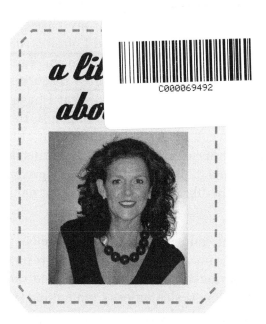

(not essential reading for diet success but may add flavour!)

- I have been devising fat loss diets for newspapers, magazines, websites and my own books for around 12 years and trialling every one of them on both myself and other 'willing victims' before they have the merest chance of 'going to print' so not only do I appreciate how hard it is to stick to a diet, lose weight and keep it off but also how important it is that any kind of fat loss diet be slotted in to a hectic and often-stressful lifestyle with minimal disruption.

- I love food, I love cooking and I love eating but am also willing to confess to being a little vain, like to look good and love being able to climb into a pair of skinny jeans without fear of an uncomfortably-tight waistband so I follow my own advice and most of the time (but certainly not all of the time!) stick to a diet that I now know, after years of trial and error, works for me.

- I cheat, I overeat, I indulge my passion for chocolate and chips (not together!) and I often struggle to hit the exercise mat or go out for a run so am regularly forced to delve into my somewhat limited resources of willpower and self-discipline. However, what I have discovered is that after a day or two of indulgence, the sooner I get back on track by dragging myself out of bed and doing some sort of exercise then concentrating on eating light for a couple of days - soup generally predominates - the greater the likelihood that no lasting damage has been done.

- I don't like counting so I don't pay heed to the number of calories I consume in a day - much more on this later. Nor do I laboriously measure portions and rarely bring out the weighing scales unless I am baking (measurements are vital for a light sponge!)

- Fortunately, I like getting out in the fresh air even when the weather is depressingly wet, windy and cold so my favourite form of exercise, cycling is my saviour. A couple of hours on my bike clears all the nonsense out of my head, helps me focus and the deep and steamy bath rich with mineral salts, the large glass of red and a bit of comedy on the radio ensures I generally come back down to earth with a smile.

- I read everything I can get my hands on with regard to diets and fat loss and try to keep up to speed with the very latest research so I can not only pass on my thoughts to my readers but also come up with new and exciting strategies to help them reach their fat loss goals.

- I like to rant and guarantee I will never hold back when it comes to giving my views on some of the crazy and sometimes dangerous weight loss tactics that are championed by those in my industry who I suspect (perhaps cynically) are only in it for the bucks.

- I love creative, young people whose passion and refusal to follow trends knows no bounds and I adore cats and can totally understand why they were worshipped as gods in ancient times - one piercing glance and you just know they are despairing of us humans and our emotionally-overburdened approach to life! I am addicted to murder mysteries and spend rather too much of my hard-earned cash downloading everything in that genre to my Kindle and I would be in seventh heaven if I were invited by some brave TV channel to pack a small bag and travel the world for weeks or months looking at traditional diets and eating habits which are sadly being lost thanks to the perceived convenience of processed, fast and junk food which seem to be doing little other than making us sick and fat!

- **NB:** I find books that are littered with links hard to handle - they ruin the flow in my view. You will note that in this book (actually, in all my books), I refer to nutritional studies, dietary experiments and the like. You can be confident that all have been well-researched but should you wish to know more, contact me through **www.fatbustforever.com** and I will happily provide the sources.

ONE MORE THING...

If you want to see pictures of all the dishes included, head to the 'Gallery' page on my website **www.fatbustforever.com** and be inspired! And, on the same page you can see me and my series of four videos explaining the principles behind the diet.

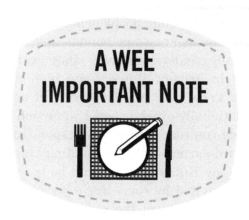

A WEE IMPORTANT NOTE

A week on a diet that focuses on fat loss and inch loss and provides sufficient good quality calories to meet our energy needs results in a loss of around...

3 POUNDS OF FAT AND 1 GALLON OF WATER

and the likelihood of keeping it off and losing more is good!

....

A week on a diet that focuses on weight loss and is low or very low on calories results in a loss of around....

1 POUND OF FAT AND 2 GALLONS OF WATER

and the likelihood of keeping it off and losing more is largely about willpower and how well we cope with hunger and cravings!

CONTENTS

A Little Bit About Me   1

Let's Talk Diets!   7

Why Super Fast?   8

Are You Ready to Super Lose?   9

The Seesaw Strategy   13

Diets Have to Be Exciting   15

Butter is Back!   16

No Time to Cook?   19

If You Are Not Hungry, Don't Eat!   20

Why No Calorie Counting?   22

Fat Loss or Weight Loss?   24

A Quick Word About Portion Size   26

The Fibre Menace   28

What's the Scoop on Fruit?   29

Chocolate is a Daily Essential!   31

Make Mine a Mint Tea   33

The Miracle Mineral   34

Feeling Tired?   35

The Exercise Question   36

Supplement Strategies   38

Before You Start   40

The Diet Plan   41

When Time is Really Tight   44

Out and About Options   46

Fats and Oils   47

Drinks   48

Recipes for Success   49

    Hot Lemon and Ginger   49

Ginger Pickle 50
Vegetables and Toppings 50
Fried Egg with Ham and Tomato 52
Poached Egg Special 53
Warm or Cold Salad 54
My Favourite Warm Salad 55
Lettuce Wraps 56
Mushroom Soup with Tofu Croutons 58
Deliciously-Light Fish Broth 60
Parcel-Baked Fish 61
Lemon Ginger Chicken 62
Tofu Towers 64
Aromatic Lamb/Beef Stew 65
Spicy Meatball Soup 66
Parsley Soup with Chicken Nuggets 68
Mackerel Magic 69
Salmon with Roasted Vegetables 70
Mexican-Style Omelette 72
Nutty Bircher Muesli 74
Scrambled Eggs on Hot Buttered Toast 75
Light Chicken Broth 76
Spinach and Watercress Soup 77
Crispy-Topped Baked Fish, Chicken or Tofu 78
Perfect Overnight Porridge 80
Thai Curry Sweet Potato Soup 81
Warm Salad with Haggis 82
Mince and Mash 83
Rice and Stuff 85
Fragrant Chicken Casserole 86
My Books, Blogs Etc. 88
Websites, Blogs 89
Copyright 91

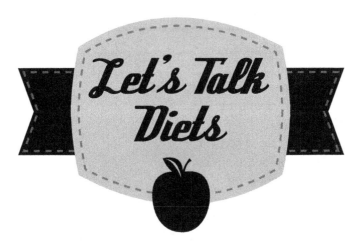

Let's Talk Diets

The wonderful thing about diets is that they generally work if you stick to them! Apart from some that champion rather dodgy tactics like taking a load of diet pills (please don't fall into that trap) or living on syrup, lemon and water for a couple of weeks, many are well-researched and don't merit the bad press they often generate.

However, sticking to a diet until we reach our fat loss goal is where many of us come unstuck. Fat loss is my subject so rather than simply skimming through the pages of every new diet that hits the headlines and critiquing them based on the thinking and/or research behind them, I try most of them out and use a very large notebook to record the experience. I devote copious pages to each diet and note down my thoughts at the end of each day. After seven days, which is usually around the time when I can ascertain whether a diet has stickability or not I review my scribblings. The purpose of this time-consuming and occasionally-gruelling exercise is not so that I can arrogantly sling mud at some of the diets that make grandiose weight loss claims - I prefer to leave that to others. No, there is method behind my obsessive attention to detail. I am continually on a quest to devise diets that deliver both fast and lasting results and that can only happen if my diets address the reasons dieters often throw in the towel. Here are the most commonly recorded:

- Hungry all the time
- Constant cravings
- Weight loss promise not achieved
- Too much shopping
- Expensive
- Foods are hard to find
- Laborious food preparation
- Too much cooking
- Meal options are bland and tasteless
- Bloating and digestive discomfort
- No energy
- Trouble sleeping
- Boring and repetitive
- Difficult to fit into work/social life

My scribbles reveal a lot about how many or how few of the above complaints are addressed by some diets and that is what excites me and permanently pushes me forward to come up with new strategies.

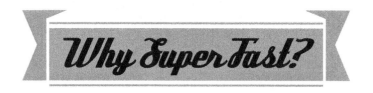

Why Super Fast?

Why not? I refuse to go along with the wide-held belief that quick fix diets don't work and also appreciate that we live in a super fast world so we want super fast results. As long as a diet positively ticks all (or most) of the above boxes and provides us with the nutrients to get through the day, improve our health and with luck, teach us a few new eating habits, I fail to understand why so much negativity surrounds the quick fix approach.

WHEN WE SEE RESULTS IN JUST A FEW DAYS WE ARE MUCH MORE LIKELY TO KEEP GOING

A couple of years ago I wrote and published my **2 Weeks in the Fast Lane** diet which continues to generate a great deal of enthusiasm. Dieters regularly report dropping a dress size in just two weeks and many continue with the basic plan and/or add a few of their own or my suggestions to keep going for many weeks thereafter. However, I am often asked to recommend a strategy for super fast fat loss before an event or a holiday or after a few weeks of overindulgence; a healthy diet that is going to see inches lost no matter how little time we have. So, here it is: my new **2 Weeks in the Super Fast Lane** diet which you can follow for anywhere between 4 and 14 days and see super fast results. Some may be able to stick to it for longer but beware of diet boredom; the dieter's nemesis. My recommendation would be to move on to my **2 Weeks in the Fast Lane** diet or my **Soup Can Make You Thin** diet, both of which present different strategies making diet boredom unlikely. You can always leap back into the super fast lane any time you wish for a few days.

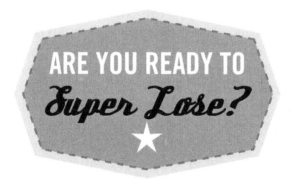

Stickability may not be a real word but to my mind it should be because when it comes to quick fix diets, if we don't stick it, we won't lose it!

Some of my diets encourage a 'mix it up and do what suits you' approach but for super fast fat loss there have to be rules. I prefer to call them strategies as that sounds altogether less prescriptive and onerous but in essence, they are still rules and if you want to shed fat fast and shave off a few inches, they have to be followed pretty closely.

Here are the most important rules with a quick explanation as to why they work for super fast fat loss. Some may go against some of the healthy eating advice you have read or heard but stick with me and you will understand why!

Go Low on Fibre. Yes, it is fabulous stuff and yes, many of us could do with upping our daily intake but few of us have the efficient digestive systems of our forebears, thanks to our now often-malnourished, Western-style diet so a too-rapid increase in fibrous foods, so often recommended in healthy diet plans can result in bloating and digestive discomfort rather than weight loss in the early stages - we have to walk before we can run and ease our way into a fabulously-healthy, fibre-rich diet.

Eat 2-3 Meals a Day. And leave 5 hours between each. The intricate relationship between the two major blood sugar hormones, insulin and glucagon is complex and delicate but put very simply, it pays to have a decent break between meals to give glucagon, the 'fat burner' the best possible opportunity to mobilise the release of stored glucose in our fat cells to be used for fuel. When we eat something every few hours or snack between meals (particularly starch and sugar-rich snacks), we continue to feed the glucose-hungry body and prompt fat storage while minimising glucagon's essential role in faster fat loss.

Drink Water When You Are Thirsty. It is crucial that we keep well-hydrated to ensure that we properly digest our food and get the maximum goodness from it but flooding the system with the often-recommended 8 glasses a day can result in us flushing out some of the vitals (vitamins and minerals that is) before they have a chance to do their vital work. What many forget to point out is that most foods contain water (yes, even meat) so if we eat a good and varied diet and have the odd cuppa here and there, 2-3 glasses are plenty unless the weather is unseasonably hot or we are doing a lot of strenuous exercise.

Drink Between Meals Not With Meals. In addition to the above, washing down every other mouthful and rushing our meals means less chewing and chewing is the first and important part of the digestive process. When we shock the stomach by sending down a mass of under-chewed, overly-wet food it struggles to break everything down and package up the goods for the next digestive process and indigestion, heartburn, belching and bloating can occur, compromising fat loss.

Make Carbs Work for You. Carbohydrate confusion reigns with conflicting advice about low carbing, no carbing, carb counting and the rest invading the minds of dieters everywhere! We don't actually need carbohydrates to survive as the body can get sufficient glucose (body sugar) from a diet rich in protein and fat, hence the appearance of so many very low carb diets since Dr Atkins first presented this theory to the masses. However, hunger and sugar cravings are common, stickability is hard and a diet which is short on the fibre and protective plant chemicals provided by fruits and vegetables is nothing short of madness, health-wise. A **seesaw approach** where fruits and vegetables are included every day but starchy carbohydrates are only included every 4 days works a great deal better, is easier to fit into a busy schedule and keeps levels of the appetite hormone, leptin working with us rather than against us. This route should not be confused with 'carb cycling', much-favoured by bodybuilders and athletes to shed body fat fast before competition (commonly known as shredding) which is way too extreme for most of us and not recommended.

11

VERY LOW CARB = VERY LOW CHANCE OF LONG TERM FAT LOSS

Have a Bit of Butter! Hallelujah, saturated fat is making a comeback! Many studies show no relationship between saturated fat intake and heart disease and there is no research into reducing saturated fat in the diet that has found that it reduces death rates. Butter is at last getting the attention it deserves and knocking chemically-altered vegetable oil concoctions off the shelves. Butter from pasture/grass-fed cows is a good source of bone-nourishing, fat busting and heart-friendly nutrients and there is simply no contest between it and the vast array of spreadable slimes on offer when it comes to taste! I also heartily endorse the inclusion of coconut oil, rich in both saturated and monounsaturated fats for cooking and spreading.

Play Smart With Fruit. Too much fructose (fruit sugar) in our diet leads to increased fat storage both on our hips, bums and tums and much more worryingly from a health point of view, around our internal organs but that in no way makes fresh fruit a no-no. Where improved digestion and super fast fat loss is concerned, you need to know which to eat and when - and no, bananas are **not** fattening!

Think Before You Breakfast. If you are not hungry first thing in the morning, don't force it down. Whilst a few studies indicate that those who don't have breakfast gain weight long term, just as many show that having your first meal of the day when you actually feel hungry leads to us reducing our food intake during the day. But, if you are one of those people who can't function without early morning nourishment, you need to 'breakfast like a king' not like a hamster - eggs are in, cereals are risky!

Have A Daily Chocolate Fix! Good quality chocolate prompts the production of both the 'reward' chemical, dopamine and the 'happy, relaxed and calm' chemical, serotonin, the fats are mostly monounsaturated, providing health benefits similar to olive oil and a little chocolate every day knocks sugar cravings on the head. More on the fabulousness of chocolate later.

Eat To Ease The Stress. Any kind of stress on the body be it emotional, physical, nutritional or physiological prompts the overactivity of the fat-storing hormone, cortisol. Magnesium, which is sadly deficient in many diets is a must for keeping cortisol levels under control, making fat loss faster and magnesium-rich foods have a super-calming effect on the digestive system.

Supplement for Success. Not a rule but those I recommend either support the digestive system, control cravings or help to accelerate the fat burning process when taken regularly and sensibly.

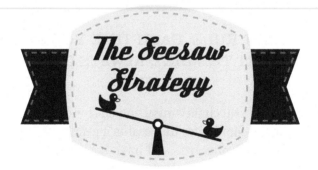

The Seesaw Strategy

Do you remember when you were young and you and your friends spent hours in the playground trying to keep the seesaw evenly balanced? Well, that's what you are going to do here. Starchy carbohydrates (bread, pasta, potatoes, beans, lentils, rice and other grains) are not the enemy to weight loss, they just have to be carefully managed. We can all cope without them for a few days but any longer than that and cravings invade - we start dreaming of buttered toast! The reason this diet includes starchy carbohydrates every fourth day is so this doesn't happen. When you know they are not off limits you don't feel deprived and miserable and the days when they are not included are a breeze.

It's simple - that's why it works. You have three 'no starch' days followed by one 'starch' day and keep repeating this four day cycle for as many days as you have decided to follow the diet. I recommend a minimum of seven days as this allows you to appreciate how easily you can fit the **seesaw strategy** into your life but sometimes emergency tactics are called for and you only have a few days before you have to slip into your favourite little black dress, skinny jeans or bikini (slimline suits, hip-hugging jeans and barely-there trunks in the boys' case). That's ok but I urge you to get back to the four day cycle just as soon as the event is over rather than taking a u-turn back to old eating habits or the pounds will pile on faster than you can say "make mine a 12 inch with everything on it"!

ONE LAST RULE: EACH TIME YOU START OR RE-START THE DIET, ALWAYS GO BACK TO DAY ONE

There are ten no starch day meal choices for days 1-3 and five starch day meal choices for day 4 plus a number of additional choices from day 5 onwards. All have been carefully created to provide maximum nourishment and include a good variety of foods that are easy to find on most supermarket/local store shelves. I have purposely kept the list of foods included reasonably short so you can plan ahead, shop ahead, repeat meals as you wish and most importantly, minimise digestive stress. If you don't digest and absorb your food efficiently, fat loss is compromised so 'tender loving care' is where it's at and that includes such comforting delights as mashed potatoes and buttered toast - yes, really!

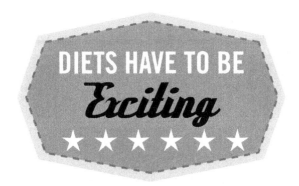

DIETS HAVE TO BE Exciting
★ ★ ★ ★ ★ ★

I love food so I want my diet (and yours) to be exciting! Having personally tested many weight loss plans and stuck, sometimes tortuously to most of them for the required amount of time I have determined that many are rather bland and somewhat repetitive. They may result in the desired weight loss but I find myself counting the days until I can return to my preferred, altogether more delicious meal choices. To lose fat, the majority of us have to make a few changes and eat less (occasionally more) than normal so it is imperative that we look forward to every meal and enjoy every bite, otherwise the whole shopping, preparation and eating process can quickly become a cheerless chore. With that in mind, I always endeavour to make my recommended meals tasty and tempting. I spend a great deal of my life playing around with ingredients and trying to come up with recipes that involve all the foods I know will help my readers get slim and stay slim and whilst some recipes may require a little more time in the kitchen, I hope you will agree that they are worth the extra effort.

AND THAT INCLUDES BUTTER!

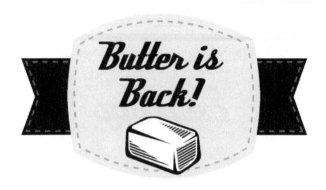

Consider the following ingredient labels:

Grass-fed Butter (unsalted)
Pasturised Cream

A Typical 'Butter Alternative'
Vegetable Oils
Water
Buttermilk
Modified Maize Starch
Salt
Emulsifiers - E471
Sunflower Lecithin
Soya Lecithin
Preservative - Potassium Sorbate
Lactic Acid
Colours - Annatto, Curcumin
Flavouring

Which looks more natural? Easy, the grass-fed butter! There is just one ingredient as opposed to a list of oils and extracts that you are likely unfamiliar with and possibly have little idea as to whether they are good or bad for your health and waistline. So, why are supermarket shelves groaning with spreads that claim everything from lowering levels of damaging cholesterol to increasing your intake of important health-enhancing nutrients and much else besides whilst discouraging you from adding a knob of butter to give your vegetables a golden glow and a little added deliciousness?

Butter has merited a great deal of adverse publicity over the years, principally because it is rich in saturated fat and the inclusion of saturated fats in our diet has long been deemed 'one to watch' and associated with raising levels of 'bad' and health-disrupting cholesterol, prompting high blood pressure, heart disease and all manner of other debilitating health conditions. But as mentioned in my intro, there is no proven relationship between saturated fat intake and heart disease and no research into reducing saturated fat in the diet has found that it reduces death rates. So where did it all go so horribly wrong and why are the diet police now, ever so quietly and almost imperceptibly backing down and beginning to hint that perhaps a little saturated fat in our diets isn't the big, bad monster they had us believing for the past 20 years or so?

Here are a few biochemical facts:

- Saturated fat forms around 50% of the membranes (protective coats) of our body cells and gives them the necessary strength and health to ensure vital nutrients enter and waste exits.

- Saturated fat plays a vital role in the health of our bones by ensuring bone-building calcium is properly absorbed.

- Saturated fat helps the body reduce levels of lipoprotein (a), a risk factor for heart disease.

- Saturated fat protects the liver from alcohol, toxins and the damage caused by the regular use of medicinal drugs.

- Saturated fat is needed for the efficient function and

repair of brain cells; the brain is made up of fats (mainly saturated) and cholesterol.

- Saturated fat enhances the immune system. When white blood cells are deficient, it hampers their ability to recognise and destroy foreign invaders such as viruses and bacteria.

- Saturated fat is needed for the proper utilisation of essential fatty acids. Health-enhancing omega-3 fats are better retained in our tissues when our diet includes saturated fats.

- Saturated fat has important antimicrobial properties; it protects us against harmful micro-organisms in the digestive tract.

- Saturated fat is essential for the production of important hormones.

- Saturated fat acts as a carrier for certain vitamins and is vital for mineral absorption.

It is the unhealthy chemically-altered fats that are found in margarines, hydrogenated vegetable oils and many processed foods that cause significant health problems plus an overabundance of sugar and refined carbohydrates which disrupt blood sugar and insulin levels that encourage fat production and storage in the body.

Processed fats are the 'ones to watch', not top-dollar butter. I am not recommending you slather it on everything but as the saying goes; a little of what you fancy... Other sources of saturated fats I include in this diet (in respectable amounts) are lean animal meats, a little dairy and coconut oil.

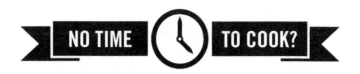

NO TIME TO COOK?

Enter the lunchbox and the wide-necked thermos flask; they are the perfect answer to ensuring we stick to a diet when we are at work or know we are going to be out and about. However, few of us lead perfect lives and days when we don't have time to plan or cook ahead or have to eat out can be hard to handle and this is where we can become a bit unstuck. For that reason, I have included 'out and about' options for both 'non starch' and 'starch' days so you know what to choose both off the shelves and when in restaurants. For the purposes of this diet, these options are geared toward getting you out of trouble occasionally but I urge you to remember that you are always going to be more in control of the diet when you prepare the meals yourself so try to plan ahead.

WHAT IF YOU DON'T LIKE SOME OF THE FOODS INCLUDED?

Unless you are very picky, this shouldn't be a problem. There are always alternatives and I am offering plenty of choices so hopefully there will be sufficient to appeal to most tastes. Having said that, this is not a diet that will suit everyone. You will find information and links at the back of the book that I encourage you to investigate should you be coeliac, diabetic, wish to 'go raw' or vegan or suspect you may have food intolerances that could be hampering your weight loss. It is also important, should you have any ongoing medical condition, be pregnant or breastfeeding or have a history of eating disorders that you consult your GP or health practitioner before embarking on any fat loss programme.

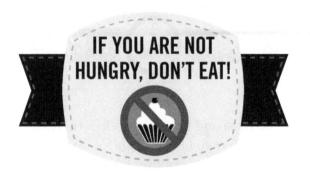

IF YOU ARE NOT HUNGRY, DON'T EAT!

This may sound like a rather obvious and simplistic piece of advice but we humans are creatures of habit and often eat at the same times each day or eat when others around us are eating which can result in us eating too much and/or too often. Conversely, it is also all-too-easy to forget to eat for hours on end when we are busy which leads to blood sugar and energy levels taking a dive; this scenario has danger written all over it for dieters as the drive to scoff whatever is nearest to hand can be overwhelming. Finding the middle ground where we only eat when we are hungry and only eat enough to satisfy our energy requirements is easier said than done but for fast and lasting fat loss is crucial. Dieters often tell me that they experience huge energy dips at certain times on certain days even though they have eaten only an hour or two previously (mid afternoon is the most common but mid morning and late evening can also be a struggle). This is where keeping a food diary for a few days can be invaluable. I have to confess I rarely come across anyone whose face lights up when I suggest a food diary which has rather a lot to do with the fact that we would rather forget the four chocolate biscuits rather than record them and see them staring back at us from the page! If I suspect nutritional deficiencies may be compromising health, I recommend a straightforward 'what you ate and when' style of diary but where fat loss is the goal I take a different and more helpful approach; a hunger diary. Every one of us is different and every day is different; work, social and domestic demands change daily, stress levels can be off the scale one day and we can be cool as cucumber the next and our hunger and appetite hormones respond accordingly. Keeping a hunger diary for a few days (preferably a week where a weekend is included) tends to reveal patterns where we can see when and why we experience energy dips and how we cope with them. By using a notebook, laptop, tablet or mobile phone and simply taking a few minutes every few hours to scribble down how you feel (in control or irritable, tired or full of beans, stressed or calm, hungry or satisfied, craving sugar/salt or merely looking for a cup of tea or a glass of water etc.) you start to see not only the times of day when energy dips occur and hunger invades but also why your current eating habits may be hindering rather than helping you achieve your fat loss goal.

As mentioned, some people are not hungry first thing in the morning but force down breakfast because it is alleged to be the 'most important meal of the day', others can't focus unless they have had some nourishment before they go out the door. The same applies to lunch and dinner; sometimes we can be ravenous around lunchtime but not at dinner and vice versa so it makes a great deal of sense to eat when you are hungry rather than eating simply because we have been programmed to have breakfast, lunch and dinner at regulated times of the day. Get off that treadmill, have a good feed at those times of the day when you know you need one to keep you firing on all cylinders and if you are not hungry, don't eat!

On this diet, I recommend 2-3 good, satisfying meals a day; some days you may need three, other days just two will work for you - determine when your really hungry times are, follow your instincts and whenever possible, don't allow the diet saboteurs (friends, family, workmates) to force you into eating just because they are. No matter how supportive they may seem, some feel the need to question or undermine your determination - they don't like it when you are shedding fat, your waistline is shrinking and you are looking good whilst they are devouring another large portion of fries!

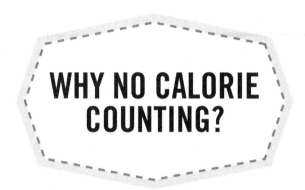

WHY NO CALORIE COUNTING?

Because this can be the rocky road to diet ruin! Please take a bit of time to read and re-read the following until they are indelibly stamped on your brain:

- There is no evidence to back up the 'calorie theory' that asserts that to lose one pound of fat we merely have to create a deficit of 3500 calories and thanks to dedicated anti-obesity researchers, slowly but surely people are beginning to understand why our obsession with calorie counting often results in weight fluctuation rather than long term fat loss. If the somewhat-simplistic principles of the 'calorie theory' were true, we would all happily shed fat weekly by sticking to a reduced calorie diet but we don't. Let's say you are a woman aged 30, weighing in at 140lbs, have a reasonably active lifestyle and you cut 500kcals per day from the recommended 2000kcals (this fits very neatly into the 3500kcals deficit mantra). Continue this for just one year and and even with the occasional blow-out on heydays and holidays, you should expect to lose around 80 pounds of fat, making you the size of a 5 year old child and probably very sick! It doesn't make mathematical sense but somehow we been hoodwinked into believing it and weight loss frustration continues to plague us.

- If your diet regularly includes junk, fast and processed foods and drinks no matter how 'low cal' the label tells you they are, you will likely put on weight and you will probably struggle to lose it no matter how many hours you pound the pavements or pump iron. The added sugars, chemically-altered fats and preservatives required to make these foods 'tasty' and give them a decent shelf life put a lot of stress on the body as it tries to metabolise what it regards as 'hard to handle' molecules. This results in the metabolic process that prompts the action of the very important fat burning hormones and enzymes being compromised.

• When we eat proper food that has had minimal or no processing and consequently has a shorter shelf/refrigerator life we not only get an abundance of energy-enhancing nutrients that haven't been messed around with but also a good package of vitamins and minerals that are so important when it comes to goading the fat burning mechanism into action.

• Going hungry for a number of hours can sometimes feel like a life-threatening emergency when we are used to regular fuelling and satisfying our growling stomachs or reversing bouts of low blood sugar-induced drowsiness. But, let's get real here, unless we are diabetic or have a medical condition where regular feeding is vital, hunger is something we can all cope with and when we get used to the odd bout here and there, isn't really that invasive. However, when we go low on calories or top-notch nourishment for days or weeks on end it can turn into not just a perceived hunger emergency but a biochemical emergency. Our super-hungry brain needs fed if we want to keep the communication lines open between it and the the millions of body cells that are looking for energy to keep the heart pumping, build bone, feed muscle, nourish our blood, protect us from disease and keep the metabolic fire burning. Poor quality and/or insufficient calories result in poor quality and insufficient energy to keep things ticking over nicely to enable us to both stay healthy and shed fat.

So, rather than counting them obsessively or reducing them drastically we need to ensure that every diet be it super fast, fast or slow and steady provides the brain and body with sufficient, good quality calories to make their day, every day.

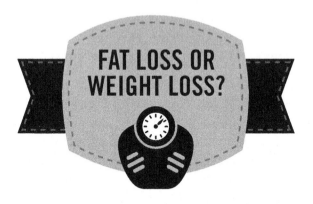

FAT LOSS OR WEIGHT LOSS?

Weighing scales should be a kitchen essential, not a bathroom accessory! Jumping on the scales every morning can lead to us throwing in the towel before we have completed the diet programme. Even when we are steadily losing inches, dropping a dress size and feeling great, dieters appear to be obsessed with what the scales say and when they don't see pounds lost, they panic. Sadly, this obsession is fuelled by weight loss stories reported daily and when similar results are not achieved we either see the diet as having failed us or us having failed the diet - hardly a lesson in positivity! I struggle to understand why pounds lost seems to be the golden ticket when in my experience most people are euphoric when they see the inches melting away without having to watch a little needle waver from left to right to determine whether they are making progress or not.

A week on a diet that focusses on fat loss and inch loss and provides sufficient good quality calories to meet our energy needs results in a loss of around 3 POUNDS OF FAT and 1 GALLON OF WATER and the likelihood of keeping it off and losing more is good.

A week on a diet that focusses on weight loss and is low or very low on calories results in a loss of around 1 POUND OF FAT and 2 GALLONS OF WATER and the likelihood of keeping it off and losing more is largely about willpower and how well we cope with hunger and cravings.

YOUR CHOICE, BUT THINK ABOUT IT!

If you find it really hard to bin the scales, try to stick to once a week (same day, first thing in the morning) and keep the following in mind when you do. Water is everywhere in the body and levels can shift at any moment for all kinds of reasons (injury, infection, menstruation, digestive stress, eating too much, eating too little, hormone imbalance and many more) so your weight - or what the scales say - can shift up or down **by anything from 2-5 pounds in a day.** But that doesn't necessarily mean you are not steadily losing fat, so if you are sticking to this diet, please don't freak out when you step on the scales; look in the mirror or check how your waistband is feeling instead and press on! Water is weighty stuff - a litre weighs in at around 4 pounds - so if your body is holding on to water (more of a problem for women than men, unfairly) it is a bit like stepping on the scales with a litre bottle in your hand - you will obviously weigh more. This diet concentrates on greatly reducing the chances of water being retained but there will always be days when levels fluctuate more than others.

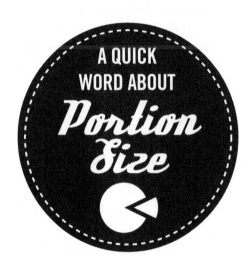

A QUICK WORD ABOUT *Portion Size*

By now it is probably crystal clear that I am not big on counting. Be it calories, pounds lost/gained or percentages of sugars, salt and fat in foods; all that counting in a bid to shed the flab is tiresome. However, I can get a bit over-zealous about portion sizes. For successful and super fast fat loss most of us have to downsize our portions, although some may have to upsize. This is not the kind of diet where you eat whatever your want for a number of days as long as you remember to semi-starve on other days. Nor is it the kind of diet where you consume way too few calories and don't meet your energy needs.

THIS IS A DIET WHERE YOU EAT REGULARLY BUT NOT TOO OFTEN AND EVERY TIME YOU EAT, YOU EAT WELL

If you have any super-slim friends who somehow or other seem to manage to stay that way you may have noticed that many of them eat more than you do but as soon as they are full, they stop eating - very irritating when you are fighting the urge to order a dessert or tidy up the bread basket! But the truth is, most of the time they really are full and couldn't stuff in another morsel because they have pigged out on food that satisfies their hunger, fills them up and most importantly, feeds their fat cells with just enough to keep them healthy and efficient but not enough to encourage them to move into super-storing mode.

To get into and stay in the fat burning zone we have to major on a strategy where food combinations, timing and portions are balanced in such a way that our fat cells become active and happy rather than lazy and lacklustre. An adult with a healthy amount of fat has around 25 to 30 billion fat cells, all of which do an amazing job of storing energy and producing important hormones but when we are overweight and continue to get 'fatter' we grow new fat cells which are simply surplus to requirement; it is estimated that the number can increase to anywhere between 75 and 200 billion! Also, a fat cell can expand to 5-6 times its original size (think of a balloon filling with water) so it is little wonder we are forced into buying bigger clothes! To get leaner, we need to halt the multiplication process and shrink the fat cells back to their 'healthy' size; this requires a bit of focus but is **not** mission impossible. The whole process centres around learning the art of eating in a way that keeps the whole metabolic process firing; only then can we expect the important hormones and enzymes that prompt stored fat to be burned for energy to work their magic.

Filling a small plate to the max is emotionally more satisfying than positioning the same amount of food on a larger plate; countless experiments reveal that all that white space may make food look great in pictures and in on-trend restaurants but leads us to believing we have eaten less than we need or want. Don't risk it! When you are eating at home and looking for super fast fat loss, pick smaller plates, bowls and mugs, use the same ones every day, fill them full to bursting and don't stop until you have hoovered the lot. It is a lot harder when you are out and about as you have little control over portion size but it pays to be a pest in restaurants. Ask for a small portion or have two starters, add a salad or vegetables and stress the need for a decent-sized portion of these, not just a bit of colour on the side and eat everything slowly. Another invaluable trick is to opt for soup. No matter what the soup of the day is, unless the weather is scorching hot, go for it. Soup fills you up fast, is satisfying and is generally a very nourishing way to ensure you don't overeat - as long as you don't make a beeline for the bread basket.

YOU MAY WANT MORE.....

This is a plan that can be followed for anywhere between **4 and 14 days**, designed in such a way that you burn fat fast and see results fast but should you wish to continue it for longer, go ahead; it won't compromise your health in any way. However, as mentioned, diet boredom can creep in despite your best efforts so make sure you mix things up a bit to keep it exciting. Alternatively, you may wish to move on to one of my other diets, **2 Weeks in the Fast Lane** or **Soup Can Make You Thin** for a while and you can come back to this diet any time you choose.

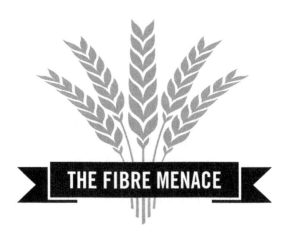

Is there is anything left to say about the importance of eating a rainbow of colourful vegetables to keep us in tip top condition? Possibly not. They pack a mighty punch nutritionally and the list of health benefits linked to including a rich variety in our diet is long and impressive. When it comes to fat loss they are also top performers and should play a major role in all diets. However, going from a diet which has been a bit bland and light on fibre for some time to one that is overflowing with vibrant colour can pose problems. It is not unusual for people who decide to embark on diets focussing on an abundance of vegetables that they are not used to eating regularly to experience stomach upsets, wind and bloating and/or suffer from nagging headaches, sleep problems and hard to manage snack attacks, all of which can be a major hindrance and extremely frustrating.

Some vegetables are easier to digest than others, dependent on their fibre content. Those that are very fibrous can take a bit of getting used to if your digestion is not up to scratch so taking it slowly is the best route. Removing the peel or tough outer layers can also help in the early stages. This diet focusses on those that are least likely to create wind, bloating and other digestive issues and with luck, after a few weeks you can hit the veg shelves with gusto and get the maximum protection from the colourful delights on offer.

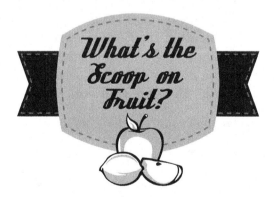

What's the Scoop on Fruit?

There is a disturbing wave of fruit-bashing flowing through nutritional channels currently. The premiss being that fruit is mainly sugar (fructose) and too much sugar in our diet leads to poor health and ever-expanding waistlines. It's hard to argue with this but there is a big difference between the effect the natural sugar in fruit has on our health and the effect of concentrated syrups and sweeteners found in many processed foods. These added sugars are everywhere and are great favourites with food manufacturers because not only do they add sweetness, which appeals to consumers' taste buds but they give products a longer shelf life because sugar is a preservative - and it's super cheap. A diet of predominantly processed food results in a sugar-laden diet, a diet of natural, 'proper' food results in a diet with a lot less sugar and this should include fruits. They are rich in fibre, some provide a reasonable amount of protein and healthy fat and I could go on for pages about the abundance of protective plant chemicals and vitamins and minerals they provide. To label fruit as 'fattening' - bananas and avocados get a lot of stick on this front - and advise dieters to limit their consumption is a trend I hope will disappear into the mist of diet myths very soon.

However, which, when and how is important where fruits are concerned. For some, but certainly not all, certain fruits can cause gas and bloating when eaten alongside other foods and as I am concentrating on a 'no bloat' strategy to aid fat loss, I recommend eating fruit on its own for the duration of the diet to minimise the risk of digestive drama. Whilst there is no snacking on this diet, fruit eaten on its own is an exception to the rule. Here are your options:

- Have fruit no less than an hour before a meal.

- Have fruit no less than 3 hours after a meal.

- Have fruit before bed if you are hungry but no less than 3 hours after your last meal.

- Have fruit during the night if you wake and can't get back to sleep.

- A mix of most fruits is fine but have banana, figs, grapes and papaya on their own or together and always have melon on its own - a mix of different melon varieties is fine.

- Before bed and during the night opt for avocado, kiwi, banana, strawberries, melon, pineapple, figs, grapes, peach, satsuma or apple as these fruits contain reasonable levels of the amino acid, tryptophan which promotes the production of the calming chemical, serotonin.

- And, remember always to chew your fruit thoroughly.

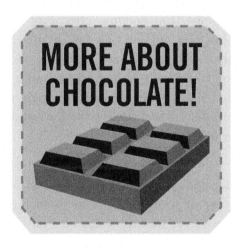

MORE ABOUT CHOCOLATE!

I can't believe I haven't mentioned chocolate for something like 33 pages...... If you don't like chocolate, there is no rule that says you have to include it but if you don't like chocolate, what's wrong with you? I recommend you have a little chocolate every day on this diet for good reason - some suggest that we should have a little chocolate every day for life but that's another story! Chocolate ticks a whole host of boxes when it comes to our health and more boxes than you might think when it comes to fat loss.

I not talking about the creamy, milky, pale stuff here, it has to be chocolate from the dark side - the type that contains at least 70% cocoa solids, better still 85%. Not only is it super-rich in plant chemicals called flavonoids which protect us against disease but it also provides a couple of protein building blocks that prompt the production of two important chemical messengers. Firstly, dopamine which makes us feel good and is often referred to as the reward chemical and secondly, serotonin which makes us feel relaxed and calm. Apart from the fact that it is hard enough to stick to a diet without the added burden of feeling miserable and deprived, there is also mounting evidence that when dopamine and serotonin levels are low, we experience appetite peaks and troughs, creating blood sugar issues and likely weight gain. Many suggest that because chocolate is rich in fat it is 'fattening' but the bulk of the fat in the dark varieties is monounsaturated fat which helps to lower levels of damaging cholesterol and reduce the amount of damaging fat we store around our organs. It is also rich in magnesium and iron which are important for fat loss and which I will discuss briefly over the next few pages.

There are various ways you can slot your chocolate fix into your day as long as you remember it's just one fix a day! Have a mini bar or around 10 squares from a bigger bar. Some find it easier to buy mini bars as putting the rest of a big bar back in the fridge for tomorrow requires a bit of discipline and doesn't always happen! Like fruit, chocolate is an exception to the 'no snacking' rule.

- One hour before one of your meals - cuts sugar cravings big time!

- With a pot of mint tea mid morning or mid afternoon - delicious combination!

- Dunked slowly and ceremonially into a mug of warmed soya milk before bed - you'll sleep like a baby!

A SUPER QUICK FIX FOR SUGAR CRAVINGS

If you are a bit of a sugaraholic, cravings can be pretty hard to handle a few days into a diet. This is where a single square of chocolate can be your salvation. When you chew and swallow food, it has to go through the digestion process before being absorbed and that can take time that you simply don't have when a sugar craving strikes but if you pop a square of chocolate under your tongue and let it dissolve slowly, the sugar will be absorbed directly into the blood stream, the urge will pass and you have only had a very small amount of sugar. It works but is not something I recommend you do too often and make sure you rinse your mouth well with water afterwards to prevent getting a dressing down from your dentist.

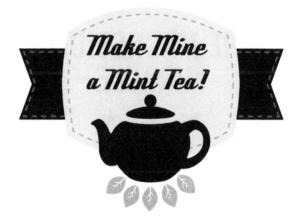

There are many herbal teas that settle the stomach, aid digestion, reduce water retention and aid sleep and it is a good idea to test some and find a few you like. To keep things simple, try some that are already mixed, come in tea bag form and have titles like 'night-time', 'relax', 'digest', 'womens', 'cleanse' etc. Some can be less than appealing to the taste buds but the secret is to let them infuse for ages -

way longer than black, green and red teas and if they are a bit too bitter, add a swirl of honey.

One that I particularly favour, which is great for the digestion, reduces flatulence fast and is very refreshing is mint - particularly delicious if you use lots of fresh leaves. When you leave them to infuse for a good 10 to 15 minutes the tea takes on a lovely sweetness (it is also good chilled). The other bonus is that restaurants, cafes etc nearly always have mint/peppermint teas on offer and a cup or two after a meal makes a great alternative to black tea or coffee when it comes to soothing the digestive tract. What many are unaware of is that mint is also a pain-killer and unlike over-the-counter medicines doesn't destroy the 'good' bacteria in the gut. There's a lot to like about mint!

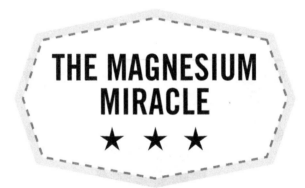

THE MAGNESIUM MIRACLE
★ ★ ★

Magnesium is required for every single cell in the body to function properly. It is sometimes referred to as the *heart-friendly* mineral as good levels are associated with a lower risk of heart disease, the *stress-friendly* mineral because it plays a major role in balancing stress hormones, the *migraine-managing* mineral as it can seriously reduce the occurrence of this debilitating condition and the *forgotten* mineral because many are ignorant of its importance, chiefly because its best mate, calcium gets more attention but deficiency is common. I call it the *smooth operator* because it has such a calming effect on the nervous system and everything works more smoothly when levels are good; reduced blood pressure, calmer and more refreshing sleep, better digestion, little or no constipation, improved physical performance with less chance of sprains and strains, a greater ability to cope with physical and emotional stress within the body and an end to menstrual cramps for many women.

There are two major reasons why magnesium is important for fat loss. One is the role it plays in keeping cortisol, the stress hormone under control which, when elevated encourages the body to store fat - particularly around the middle. The other is in the production of a hormone called adiponectin that regulates how fat is stored within the body. When we are overweight its ability to function is reduced so fat stores increase but when there is plenty of magnesium available it leaps into gear, encouraging fat to be burned.

Furthermore, when magnesium levels are low our ability to process fluids is compromised which means that fluids build up in the system and cause water retention - a real fat loss adversary as discussed. This diet is rich in foods that provide magnesium and I also suggest a supplement which helps to ensure levels are optimal.

FEELING TIRED? IRON THINGS OUT

One of the most common complaints I hear when people leap into a new diet and a slightly more vigorous exercise programme is lack of energy. The mind is willing, dogged determination is in plentiful supply but the body doesn't appear to be able to keep up. Almost all of the cells in our body burn dietary calories to create energy through a process that requires the mineral, iron. When iron stores get low, it gets harder by the day to stick to a plan.

So, how do you know if you are short of iron? Blood loss is the most common cause of iron deficiency so women who have heavy periods are particularly at risk. Common symptoms other than lack of energy include:

Pale skin
Weakness
Shortness of breath
Dizziness or lightheadedness
Cold hands and feet
Brittle nails
Fast heartbeat
An uncomfortable tingling or crawling feeling in your legs

Dietary iron comes in two forms; heme iron found in animal flesh which is easily absorbed within the body and non-heme iron found in plant foods but needs good levels of stomach acid and vitamin C to assist in its absorption. This diet is rich in both but if symptoms persist, get your iron levels checked out by your GP or health practitioner as you may require a supplemental boost.

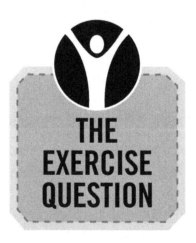

THE EXERCISE QUESTION

Which type of exercise burns fat faster? Should it be 10 minutes of pumping iron daily, half an hour of pounding the pavements 3-4 times a week, embarking on a punishing military-style training programme or doing lots of 'hot' yoga? There is no simple answer here but experts are largely in agreement that building and maintaining muscle results in us looking leaner, feeling fitter and staying healthier plus an increase in lean body mass over time is generally accompanied by a decrease in fat mass. The temptation to build muscle fast in a bid to bust fat can be strong but the likelihood of injury is often greater so best advice is to embark on some type of resistance exercise and adopt a little and often strategy in the early stages. By using dumbbells, exercise machines, your own body weight, bottles of water, elastic tubing, ankle and wrist weights or exercise bricks, muscles are strengthened by pitting each group against a force (resistance). To develop a muscle you must work all the fibres within it which means pushing them to their limit for short periods of time, resting them briefly then repeating the process. You work with a weight that is heavy enough so that the last few repetitions become difficult to perform - this is not the kind of exercise where you chat to a friend while you work out, it requires concentration and determination!

Recommendations vary but generally 10-20 minutes, every other day is a good goal and it's never too late to start. In one study of elderly men and women (average age 87) who lifted weights three times a week for ten weeks, muscle strength increased by a staggering 113% on average. This improvement in strength enabled them to walk 12% faster than before, climb 28% more stairs and lose excess body fat. On 'rest' days, get your heart pumping, expand the network of blood vessels that allow nutrients to be absorbed into body tissues and help to clear waste products from the food burning process by going for a brisk walk or light jog.

If you wish to learn more about resistance/strength training, search the internet, buy a book that covers this type of programme in detail or enlist the services of a personal trainer who practices the principles.

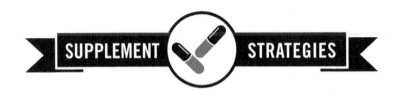

I rarely encourage anyone to supplement their diet before getting their diet right; it can be a hit or miss affair where we are often in the dark about nutrient deficiencies and can end up clutching at expensive straws. I am, however a fan of a multivitamin and mineral, particularly in the winter months; it can be hard to keep the immune system sufficiently strong and fight off every virus and bug that threatens us plus we seem to have to cope with so much more stress when the daylight hours are short. It may well be psychological but few of us feel at our absolute best at this time of the year and a good multi can provide extra insurance. My advice is always to buy the best you can afford and go for recognised and respected brands. I don't have 'relations' with any supplement companies but if you would like to know more about those that get my vote, please don't hesitate to contact me through my website, www.fatbustforever.com

Where fat loss is the goal, the market is littered with products that may improve digestion, cut cravings or accelerate fat burning and if used sensibly, there are some that can help when you are following a healthy and nutritious plan. None are essential to the plan but here are three of my favourites which you may wish to consider:

Calma-C: provides good levels of bone-building, heart-friendly and fat busting calcium with a good helping of magnesium, well-respected for its 'relaxing' properties. It also provides a boost of vitamin C which, because it is a water soluble vitamin needs to be continually topped up, particularly in the darker months to keep the immune system strong. Calma-C is a powder which can be stirred into warm water and taken an hour or so before bedtime to help relax the whole body, ensure that vital nutrients are ferried to where they are needed and promote a restorative and uninterrupted night's sleep. It is available from Higher Nature, www.highernature.co.uk and also through Amazon. There are many similar powdered products available globally. Start with a small nightly dose and build up to what is known as 'bowel tolerance' - magnesium can have an overly-relaxing effect but you will quickly know how much works for you!

Glutamine: This amino acid (part of a protein) both feeds and helps to repair the cells in the digestive tract making them stronger and better able to efficiently absorb the nutrients that aid fat burning and are vital to not only improved digestive health but better all-round health. There is also substantial evidence that glutamine helps control cravings, particularly for starchy foods and is associated with a reduction in appetite. It is available from quality suppliers in both capsule and powder form but my favourite is Biocare's L-Glutamine Powder which is available both directly from their website www.biocare.co.uk and through Amazon. A good trick is to dissolve the recommended daily dose in a small bottle of water in the morning and take regular sips throughout the day.

Krill Oil: A brilliant source of Omega 3 essential fatty acids which are essential for not only brain and heart health but also for modulating appetite and ensuring that we have the required energy and focus to stick to a diet plan. In nutritional terms, the word 'essential' means we can't make these fats within the body so have to get them from our diet. Krill is also rich in astaxanthin, the protective plant chemical which is derived from the algae these tiny fish feed on which has been shown to increase the usage of stored fat as an energy source. Udo Erasmus does an excellent product, **O-Krill 3** available through his websites, www.udoschoicekrill.com and www.udoschoice.co.uk and also through Amazon.

A FEW THINGS TO DO BEFORE YOU START

For maximum fat loss in a relatively short space of time you must follow the diet as closely as possible - a little forward planning will make this much easier. They say busy people have the most time (feel free to challenge this!) but if you can, find half an hour every evening to quickly run through how you are going to fit the diet into tomorrow and plan accordingly. This strategy seriously reduces the chances of you being stuck in a situation where you are hungry, none of your meal options are available and you end up grabbing some sort of sugary, starchy, diet-unfriendly snack.

• Decide on which meals you want to include and get the suggested foods into the fridge/freezer/cupboard.

• Make sure you have your chosen seasonings, toppings, butters, oils and drink options in stock.

• Try and find time to make the soups and stews you wish to include and refrigerate/freeze in portions. Each recipe indicates how many servings it provides so plan ahead and spend minimal time in the kitchen.

• Have your last meal of the day on the day before you start no later than 7.30pm and have Calma C (if using) before bed to 'cool the jets' and aid a good night's sleep.

• If you know you are going to be eating out at any stage while you are on the plan, have a look online at the menu beforehand, decide what you are going to have and stick to it.

• Never underestimate the fabulousness of soup to get you out of trouble. It is filling, fast and widely available so when hunger beckons and you haven't planned ahead, make it your first choice.

THE GREATER VARIETY OF FOODS YOU EAT, THE MORE ESSENTIAL NUTRIENTS YOU GET AND THE MORE ESSENTIAL NUTRIENTS YOU GET THE GREATER LIKELIHOOD OF FASTER FAT LOSS

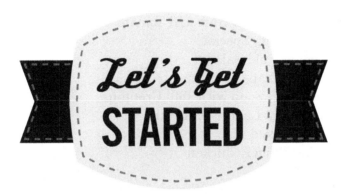

Start with days 1-4 (three non starch days followed by one starch day), move on to days 5, 6, 7 (non starch) then day 8 (starch) and continue for as many days as you wish. Should you 'fall off the wagon' at any stage, get back on track as quickly as possible, go back to day one and start over.

Every day:
- Have a mug of **hot lemon and ginger** first thing in the morning (see recipe).
- Have a spoonful of **ginger pickle** before each meal (optional - see recipe).
- Have 2-3 good-sized meals.
- Leave 5 hours between each meal.
- Drink 2-3 large glasses of water plus recommended drinks between meals but not with meals.
- Eat fruit on its own one hour before or 3 hours after a meal.
- Use butter from grass-fed cows for cooking and spreading plus other fat and oil recommendations.

- Have your last meal of the day a minimum of 3 hours before bed.
- Have your chocolate 'fix' and take your supplements (both optional).

Days 1-3
(see recipes)
- Fried Eggs with Ham and Tomato
- Poached Egg Special
- Warm or Cold Salad
- Lettuce Wraps
- Mushroom Soup with Tofu Croutons
- Deliciously-Light Fish Broth
- Parcel-Baked Fish
- Lemon Ginger Chicken
- Tofu Towers
- Aromatic Lamb/Beef Stew

Day 4
(see recipes)
- Nutty Bircher Muesli
- Scrambled Eggs on Toast
- Light Chicken Broth
- Spinach and Watercress Soup
- Crispy-Topped Baked Fish, Chicken or Tofu

Days 5-7, 9-11, 13-15, 17-19......
(see recipes)
- **All the choices from days 1-3**
- Spicy Meatball Soup
- Parsley Soup with Chicken Nuggets
- Mackerel Magic
- Salmon with Roasted Vegetables
- Mexican-Style Omelette

Days 8, 12, 16, 20.....
(see recipes)
- **All the choices from day 4**

- Perfect Overnight Porridge
- Thai Curry Sweet Potato Soup
- Warm Salad with Haggis
- Mince and Mash
- Rice and Stuff
- Fragrant Chicken Casserole

SUGGESTIONS FOR DAYS 1 - 4

You may wish to follow these suggestions to get you started. Alternatively, do your own thing and devise your own plan to suit your timetable. Choose no fewer than 2 and a maximum of 3 meals each day dependent on how hungry you are.

DAY 1 (no starch)
- Fried Eggs with Ham and Tomato
- Mushroom Soup with Tofu Croutons
- Lemon Ginger Chicken

DAY 2 (no starch)
- Deliciously-Light Fish Broth
- Warm or Cold Salad
- Aromatic Lamb/Beef Stew

DAY 3 (no starch)
- Lettuce Wraps
- Poached Egg Special
- Tofu Towers **or** Parcel-Baked Fish

DAY 4 (starch)
- Light Chicken Broth **or** Spinach and Watercress Soup
- Scrambled Eggs on Toast **or** Nutty Bircher Muesli
- Crispy-Topped Baked Fish, Chicken or Tofu

WHEN TIME IS <u>REALLY</u> TIGHT AND DESPERATE MEASURES ARE REQUIRED

If you only have 3 days before an event or a holiday and minimal kitchen time available you can select just a few quick 'non starch' dishes and repeat them. Here's what I do when I am up against the clock and crazy busy. 2 good meals a day are plenty with the recommended fruits, drinks, supplements and of course, chocolate thrown into the mix. Works for me and many others who find themselves in similarly-desperate straights - try it!

EVERY DAY

First thing
20 minutes of resistance exercise followed by a mug of **Hot Lemon and Ginger**, a multivitamin and mineral supplement, a Krill oil capsule and a large glass of water

Between 10am and 11am
1 teaspoon **Ginger Pickle** followed by a **Warm Salad** (very easy to transport)

Around 2pm
A mug of green tea or miso soup (keep sachets in your handbag/desk drawer) and another Krill oil capsule

Between 3pm and 5pm
A couple of pieces of fruit (apples, pears, plums or berries are good at this time of the day) and a large glass of water

Between 6pm and 8pm
1 teaspoon **Ginger Pickle** followed by **Parcel-Baked Fish** or **Lemon Ginger Chicken** with a selection of steamed or microwaved greens or a green salad

If time allows
Brisk walk or jog for 20 minutes

Before Bed
A mug of warm, non-dairy milk (soya, rice, almond, oat) and a small bar of dark chocolate and/or **Calma-C** dissolved in water

Throughout the Day
Regular sips of **glutamine** powder dissolved in a bottle of water

If you have a 4th day before you have to 'perform', repeat the above or make it a 'starch' day by substituting the **Nutty Bircher Muesli** or **Perfect Overnight Porridge** for your first meal of the day and the **Crispy-Topped Baked Fish, Chicken or Tofu** for the second.

NOW THIS IS IMPORTANT!
After your 3-4 days of super-diligence, try to stick to as many of the super fast lane 'rules' as possible even when a bit of overindulgence may be on the cards. You are unlikely to see much in the way of fat or inches piling back on as long as you keep the **super fast strategies** in mind. Make it your chosen way of eating and you will be in charge with improved digestion, minimal water retention, regular fat burning and continued inch loss until you reach your goal.

IF YOU HAVEN'T PLANNED AHEAD AND HAVE TO BE OUT AND ABOUT

These options are not recommended for days 1 to 4 but may be included occasionally thereafter when you are forced to 'grab and go' or social/work engagements are unavoidable.

NON STARCH DAYS
(bread, pasta, noodles, beans, lentils, potatoes, rice and other grains **should not be included in any meals**)

- Lean bacon, poached or scrambled eggs, grilled tomatoes and mushrooms.
- Scrambled eggs with smoked salmon or cooked ham.
- Omelette or frittata with meat/poultry, vegetables and/ or cheese.
- Soup: meat/poultry/game, fish/shellfish or miso. Try to make sure they have plenty of vegetables and avoid creamy soups.
- Cold or warm salads with lean meat/poultry, fish/ shellfish or tofu and lots of raw/cooked vegetables. Go easy on ready-made dressings or do without.
- Roasted, grilled or poached meat, poultry, game, fish, shellfish, tofu, quorn with at least 3 vegetables on the side or a good-sized salad.

STARCH DAYS
(bread, pasta, noodles, beans, lentils, potatoes, rice and other grains **may be included in meals** but make sure they don't dominate)

- Scrambled or poached eggs on chunky, chewy, buttered brown toast with a couple of rashers of lean bacon on the side.
- French toast (eggy bread) topped with grilled mushrooms.
- Baked potatoes or sweet potatoes filled with meat, poultry or seafood and vegetables/salad and topped with

yoghurt, tzatziki, hummus, cottage cheese, guacamole or salsa (avoid fillings with mayonnaise).

- Soup: meat/poultry/game, fish/shellfish or miso. Try to make sure they have plenty of vegetables and avoid creamy soups.
- Cold or warm salads with lean meat/poultry, fish/shellfish or tofu and lots of raw/cooked vegetables. Go easy on ready-made dressings or do without.
- Roasted, grilled or poached meat, poultry, game, fish, shellfish, tofu, quorn with at least 3 vegetables on the side or a good-sized salad.

FATS AND OILS RECOMMENDED

For spreading:
- Grass/pasture-fed butter.
- Coconut oil or butter.
- Nut butters: peanut, cashew nut, hazelnut, almond, macadamia, pistachio, pecan, walnut (preferably organic, always sugar-free)
- Seed butters: pumpkin, sesame, sunflower, flax/linseed (preferably organic, always sugar-free)

For cooking:
- Grass/pasture-fed butter mixed with olive or avocado oil for frying and sauteeing.
- Coconut oil for frying and sauteeing.

- Olive or avocado oil for roasting vegetables or basting meat or fish.

For drizzling over cooked vegetables, salads, soups and stews:
- Nut and seed oils: walnut, peanut, pistachio, avocado, olive, pumpkin, sesame, coconut - experiment and discover the added extra oils give to so many dishes!
- Grass/pasture-fed butter: a knob of butter melted over steamed vegetables is hard to beat!
- Truffle oil: ridiculously-expensive and quite strong-tasting so a little goes a long way but a mere drizzle catapults many everyday savoury dishes into totally fabulous mode in my view!

NB: top quality butters and oils should be kept in the fridge and/or in the dark (go with the manufacturers recommendations) and they don't have a long shelf-life so experiment with just one or two at a time and decide which ones you like best rather than stocking up and having to pour good money down the drain because they are past their 'use by' date.

DRINKS RECOMMENDED

- Water: predominantly still and occasionally sparkling.
- Coconut water.
- Coffee: small, dark and bitter made from fresh beans

(no milk and sugar).

- Tea: Black, red, green, herb, fruit (no milk and sugar).
- Juices: fresh fruit, watered down 50:50 and fresh vegetable.
- Miso: sachets, pastes or freshly made.
- Hot chocolate and cocoa made with dark (preferably organic) chocolate/cocoa bean granules and almond, soy, rice or coconut milk.

RECIPES
(every day)

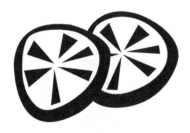

Hot Lemon and Ginger

makes 1 serving

The secret here is to make it before you shower and let it cool a little before sipping while you get ready for the day ahead.

Method
- Boil the kettle, put 1 or 2 tablespoons of freshly-squeezed lemon or lime juice in a mug (the stuff that comes in bottles is fine), grate in some peeled fresh root ginger (you can peel it, cut it into chunks, freeze and grate straight from frozen), add boiling water, stir well, leave to cool a little while you have your shower and sip while you are getting dressed.

Ginger Pickle

makes enough for around 4 days

There is nothing like ginger when it comes to calming the digestive system and if you are one of those poor souls who suffers from travel sickness, this pickle works wonders!

Ingredients
1cm piece of fresh root ginger, peeled
4 tablespoons fresh lemon juice
1 tablespoon honey (preferably Manuka)
2 tablespoons boiling water
Pinch of salt

Method
- Finely grate the ginger, put it in a jar, pour over the lemon juice, stir in the honey, water and salt, put the lid on and store in the fridge. Shake or stir before using and have 1 teaspoon before each meal.

Vegetables on the Side

It is important to get a good selection of fresh vegetables into your day, every day but as mentioned, some can be harder to digest than others so to ease the stress (from both a digestive and time perspective), focus predominantly on the following. Naturally, you reap the maximum nutritional benefits when they are eaten immediately but if time is not on your side you can 'prepare/cook and refrigerate' up to 24 hours beforehand, allowing you to pack them up, take them to work the next day and heat through or have them cold.

Steam, microwave, grill, roast or parcel-bake your vegetables or eat them raw in salads (grated carrots and courgettes are a great salad secret) and add a bit of extra zing with the recommended toppings.

Asparagus (stems peeled)
Aubergine/Eggplant

Avocado
Bok Choi (pak choi)
Carrots (peeled)
Celery (peeled)
Chillies (all types)
Courgette/Zucchini
Cucumber
Fresh herbs
Garlic
Leek
Lemongrass
Lettuce (all types)
Mangetout (snow peas)
Mushrooms (all types)
Mustard Cress (garden cress)
Olives (all types)
Onions (all types)
Peppers (red, yellow, orange)
Spinach
Sugar Snap Peas
Tomatoes
Watercress

Toppings

Lemon/lime juice and zest
Ground peppers and spices
Soy, Worcestershire, anchovy, fish, sweet chilli sauces
Toasted nuts and seeds
Nut and seed oils
Flavoured vinegars
Grated coconut
Finely grated hard cheeses

RECIPES
(no starch days)

Fried Eggs with Ham and Tomato
makes 1 serving

Once upon a time 'bacon and eggs' was regarded as a health-disrupting, only-on-a-sunday breakfast treat but happily, no more... Have this quick and easy combo first thing in the morning or whenever the mood takes you and say goodbye to sugary cereals for good.

Ingredients
½ tablespoon coconut or olive oil (or a mix of both)
2 medium free range eggs
2 thin slices Parma or other 'cured' ham
1 medium fresh tomato, halved
Freshly ground black pepper

Method
- In a small to medium-sized saute pan, heat the oil over a medium heat until hot then add the tomato halves, flesh side down and cook for a few minutes then push them to the side of the pan.

- Add the cured ham slices, let them sizzle for a minute or two before moving them to the side and cracking the eggs into the remaining space (turn the heat down if they start spluttering).

- As the eggs cook, keep basting them with the oil using a spoon and tilting the pan slightly.

- Once the eggs are cooked to your liking, season the eggs and tomato lightly with pepper (you are unlikely to need salt as the ham is 'salty') then lift all the ingredients onto a warmed plate with a slotted spoon or fish slice and dig in.

Poached Egg Special

makes 1 serving

There's something about slicing through a perfectly-cooked poached egg that is hard to match on the indulgence front. Make this combo once and you will be hooked!

Ingredients

½ tablespoon coconut or olive oil
1 large 'beef' mushroom, stem removed and top peeled
1 large free range egg
A handful of fresh baby spinach leaves
½ avocado, stone out, peeled and sliced
2 thin slices smoked ham or smoked salmon
Sea salt and freshly ground black pepper

Method

• Warm the oil in a shallow pan over a medium heat then saute the mushroom for around 5 minutes, turning regularly until well-browned and cooked through.

• Remove from the heat, turn the mushroom gill side up, lightly season, place the spinach leaves on top and cover with a lid or foil to keep warm (this allows the spinach to wilt a little).

• Bring a small pan of water to the boil, turn it down to barely bubbling, give it a good swirl with a whisk then crack the egg into the middle of the vortex and cook for 3 minutes before removing with a slotted spoon and placing it on a few sheets of kitchen towel to absorb excess water.

• Place the mushroom/spinach on a warmed serving plate followed by the sliced avocado, ham or smoked salmon and finally the egg, season to taste and eat immediately.

• This also works well with scrambled egg if you find poaching eggs a bit of a hit or miss affair!

Warm or Cold Salad

makes 1 serving

I love a challenge and when people tell me they find salads boring I shift into passionate mode! Salads shouldn't just be about chewing and crunching your way through a jungle of greens - the opportunities are endless and the more you experiment, the more quickly you can throw your favourite combinations together.

Base - all kinds of lettuce leaves, spinach leaves, watercress, bok choi, mustard cress, finely sliced celery, spring onions, salad onions, fresh herbs.

Next - tomatoes, cucumber, grated carrot, grated courgette, sliced peppers, sugar snap peas, mangetout, sliced chillies, avocado, baby asparagus, sliced mushrooms, olives, roasted vegetables, sauteed leeks or aubergine.

Consider - cold cooked chicken or turkey, cold sliced duck or game, lean cooked meats, hard cheeses (cubed, sliced or grated), feta cheese, goats cheese, cottage cheese, cooked peeled prawns, flaked fish, anchovies, sardines, fresh or tinned tuna, crab or salmon, sliced or chopped boiled egg.

To Finish - dress with a mix of some of the following: extra virgin olive oil, nut or seed oil, lemon/lime juice, flavoured vinegars, sea salt flakes, ground black pepper, soy sauce, natural yoghurt or cottage cheese, wholegrain mustard, crushed garlic or ginger, drizzle of honey, spoonful of creamed horseradish, spoonful of tzatziki, shake of chilli or curry powder, Worcester sauce, Tabasco, tomato puree.

Make it hot - use all the suggestions above but throw in some hot food for variety - chicken, prosciutto, lean lamb, chunks of minced beef, grilled fish and shellfish (tuna, mackerel, sardines, anchovies, prawns, scallops etc), roasted peppers and other vegetables, sautéed onion slices, warm freshly boiled eggs or a perfect runny poached egg, steamed vegetables and/or warm your dressing very gently and mix through your salad at the last minute.

NB: If you are taking a salad to work or you are out and about, keep the dressing separate and add just before devouring.

One of My Favourite Warm Salads
makes 1 serving

Ingredients
1 tablespoon pine nuts
1 tablespoon olive or avocado oil
½ red pepper, de-seeded and finely sliced
4 spring onions, trimmed and finely sliced
1 skinless chicken breast, carved into bite-sized slices
Crunchy lettuce leaves
Baby spinach leaves
Cucumber, peeled, seeds removed and thinly sliced
Carrot, peeled and grated
Courgette, wiped and grated
Large tomato, sliced or quartered
½ avocado, stoned, peeled and sliced

For the dressing:
3 tablespoons extra virgin olive oil
½ tablespoon white wine vinegar or lemon juice
1 teaspoon coarse grain or Dijon mustard
A pinch of sea salt
Freshly ground pepper

Method

- Toast the pine nuts in a frying pan over a medium heat until golden.

- Saute the peppers and spring onions in the oil until soft and slightly caramelised around the edges then remove with a slotted spoon and keep warm.

- Add the chicken to the remaining oil and saute gently until cooked through but still juicy.

- Mix all the dressing ingredients in a small pan or microwaveable dish and very gently heat through.

- Meanwhile, load the lettuce, spinach, cucumber, grated carrot and coriander into a salad bowl (be generous!)

- Top the salad with the hot onions and peppers followed by the hot chicken and finally the tomato, avocado and pine nuts.

- Drizzle the warm dressing over the whole dish but don't soak it, sit yourself down and enjoy.

Lettuce Wraps

Big crunchy lettuce leaves are the perfect vehicle for a 'no starch' style sandwich or two (or three or four!) I like to have all the ingredients to hand in bowls or plates and wrap as I go rather than creating neat little designer packages but it's up to you. Here are a few delicious combinations to try or you can just make up your own dependent on what's in stock.

- Tinned salmon, chopped boiled egg, sliced mixed olives, sliced avocado, sliced cucumber, natural yoghurt, lemon juice and a good dash of smoked paprika powder.

- Cold or hot sliced chicken, sauteed onions, garlic and ginger, sliced avocado, vinaigrette dressing and toasted walnuts.

- Parma ham, sauteed mushrooms, grilled or fresh tomato, scrambled egg or sliced boiled egg and Worcester sauce - breakfast in a wrap!

- Cooked minced beef or lamb, fresh mint leaves, fresh coriander, sauteed onion and red chilli pepper and fish sauce (nam plah).

- Firm tofu cubes sauteed until crisp in flavoured oil, sauteed onions, garlic, ginger and lemongrass, natural yoghurt, lime juice and toasted sesame seeds.

- Sliced beef (hot or cold), tzatziki, toasted flaked almonds, lots of fresh mint and a drizzle of honey.

- Hot or cold cooked prawns, sauteed garlic, red or yellow pepper, ginger and lemongrass, lots of fresh coriander, lime juice, natural yoghurt and toasted peanuts.

- Hot or cold cooked chicken or turkey, sauteed spring onions and yellow peppers, grated hard cheese, freshly chopped parsley and toasted flaked almonds.

- Minute steak or fillet steak, grilled and finely sliced, coarse grain mustard, sweet chilli sauce, sauteed mushrooms and spring onions, toasted cashew nuts.

- Fresh prawns or crabmeat, cucumber, chopped boiled egg, yoghurt and toasted pine nuts.

- Tinned tuna, coarse grain mustard, lime/lemon juice, anchovy sauce, sliced tomato and Greek yoghurt.

Wrap Tips:
- Don't season with salt and pepper until you have had your first bite - may not be required.

- Always use a tasty, crunchy lettuce (cos, romaine and little gem are my choices) - iceberg may create a nice neat parcel but tastes of virtually nothing!

- A few toasted nuts and/or seeds add a very desirable extra crunch - keep a selection in the fridge ready for whenever you fancy a bit of wrapping.

Mushroom Soup with Tofu Croutons

makes 2 generous or 3 small servings

A rich, dark and tasty mushroom soup is hard to beat when it comes to filling you up and providing a wealth of goodness and for those who struggle with tofu (I include myself here!), these croutons will convert you overnight - delightful on their own and great in a soup, stew or salad.

Ingredients

For the croutons:
1 thick slice firm tofu (around 2-3cm)
2 teaspoons cornflour
Sea salt
Cayenne pepper
1 tablespoon olive oil

For the soup:
20g mixed dried mushrooms
1 tablespoon olive or coconut oil
1 leek, cleaned, green leaves removed and white part very finely sliced
4 fresh chestnut mushrooms, cleaned and thinly sliced
1cm piece fresh ginger, peeled and grated
1 clove garlic, crushed
250ml vegetable stock
2 tablespoons soy sauce or tamari
1 tablespoon rice wine vinegar or lemon juice
1 large handful fresh spinach, rinsed

Method
- Preheat the oven to 200C/400F/Gas Mark 6.

- Pat the tofu dry with plenty of kitchen paper before cutting into bite-sized cubes.

- Put the cornflour in a bowl, add a pinch of salt and a good sprinkling of cayenne pepper before adding the tofu cubes and the oil. Toss until all the cubes are well-coated, lay on a non-stick baking tray and pop on a medium shelf in the oven. Bake for 30 minutes, turning regularly or until the cubes are nice and crunchy. You can make the croutons up to 24 hours before and keep them in a sealed bag and simply reheat in the oven.

- While the croutons are baking, place the dried mushrooms in a bowl, cover with boiling water and leave to soak.

- Warm the oil in a soup pot, add the leeks and saute over a medium heat until soft.

- Add the fresh mushrooms, ginger and garlic and cook for a further 5 minutes.

- Remove the dried mushrooms from the water (reserving the soaking liquid), roughly slice them, add to the pot and continue to saute for a few minutes before adding 5 tablespoons of the soaking liquid and the stock to the pot.

- Bring to the boil then reduce the heat before adding the soy sauce, vinegar and chilli paste and keep simmering for a further 5 minutes.

- Add the spinach and stir continuously until the spinach has wilted.

- Taste and add more soy sauce, vinegar or lemon juice if desired before serving topped with the tofu croutons.

Deliciously-Light Fish Broth

makes 2 generous or 3 small servings

I make this at least once a week because it's quick, delicious and so goddamned healthy! The fish, fruit de mer mix, bean mix and fish stock are always in the freezer, the fish sauce is in the cupboard and whenever I am using leek and celery for another dish I simply slice up a bit of extra, freeze it and I'm good to go with this soup after a rather frenetic day.

Ingredients

1 tablespoon olive oil
½ leek, washed, most of the dark green leaves removed and white part very finely sliced
½ stick celery, trimmed, peeled and very finely sliced
650ml homemade or bought fish stock
5 teaspoons fish sauce (nam plah)
6 tablespoons frozen pea and bean mix (peas, broad beans and green beans)
1 large or 2 small frozen white fish fillets (haddock, cod etc)
1 bag frozen 'fruit de mer' mix (prawns, mussels, scallops, squid)
White pepper

Method

· If your fish stock is frozen, defrost in the microwave or over a very gentle heat.

· Take the white fish out of the freezer and allow to slightly defrost until you can cut it into bite-sized chunks.

· Meanwhile, warm the oil in a soup pot and very gently saute the leeks and celery until tender but still with a slight 'bite' (don't let them brown).

· Add the fish stock, bring to the boil, reduce the heat, add the fish sauce and simmer for 5 minutes.

· Add the pea/bean mix and continue to simmer until

they are all tender (around 4 - 5 minutes).

- Add the frozen white fish chunks and the 'fruit de mer' mix (around 6 scallops, 6 mussels, 6 prawns and 6 pieces squid).

- Simmer gently in the broth until all the fish is cooked (around 8 - 10 minutes).

- Before serving, check the seasoning, adding a little white pepper and another splash of fish sauce if required.

Parcel-Baked Fish
makes 1 serving

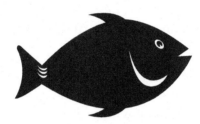

Fish was born to be baked in a parcel. All the juices meld together creating a delicious, quick and super-healthy meal. Get friendly with your local fishmonger, buy fish and vegetables in season and add herbs and spices to sharpen things up. This is one of my favourites.

Ingredients
1 white fish fillet of choice
1 generous handful of fresh spinach leaves
1 small onion, peeled and very finely sliced into rings
6 fresh asparagus tips
1 tomato, sliced
1 small red chilli, de-seeded and finely sliced (optional)
1 tablespoon fresh parsley or coriander leaves, chopped
2 teaspoons lemon juice

2 teaspoons olive oil
Sea salt and freshly ground black pepper

Method
- Preheat the oven to 200C/400F/Gas Mark 6.

- Lay out one piece of aluminium foil about 12-14" square and place the spinach on it.

- Lay the fish fillet on the bed of spinach followed by the onion, asparagus, tomato, chilli (is using) and herbs.

- Drizzle the lemon juice and olive oil over and season lightly with salt and pepper.

- Fold the foil to create a parcel, leaving plenty of space around the contents, place on a baking sheet and bake for around 25 minutes or until the fish is cooked and the juices run clear.

- Timing will depend on the thickness of the fish fillet so take a peek after 25 minutes. Be careful when opening the foil as hot steam will escape.

- When cooked, lift the contents of the parcel onto a warmed plate and spoon over the delicious juices.

Lemon Ginger Chicken
makes 1 serving

This was an experiment that really worked! The cool, creamy avocado topping married with the heat of the ginger and lemon grass and the sharpness of the lemon and vinegar takes the succulent chicken fillets into a whole new place.

Ingredients
3 skinless mini chicken fillets
1 tablespoon olive or coconut oil
1 red onion, peeled and finely sliced
1 celery stick, peeled and finely sliced

2 large tomatoes, skinned, de-seeded and chopped or a small can (200g) chopped tomatoes, sieved to remove the liquid
1 teaspoon minced ginger
1 teaspoon lemon grass paste
1 tablespoon balsamic vinegar
1 heaped tablespoon fresh coriander leaves, roughly chopped
Sea salt and freshly ground black pepper
½ ripe avocado, stoned, peeled and roughly chopped
2 teaspoons lime or lemon juice
Chilli powder (hot or mild)

Method
- Preheat the oven to 200C/400F/Gas Mark 6.

- Place the chicken fillets on a piece of baking foil large enough to form a loose parcel, lightly season, add a good splash of oil, scrunch all the edges of the foil together, place in an oven-proof baking dish and bake for 8-10 minutes or until the chicken is cooked through and the juices run clear then set aside, covered.

- Warm the oil in a small saute pan, add the onion and celery and cook gently until they are soft but not browned.

- Add the tomato, ginger, lemon grass and vinegar, stir well and continue to cook over a medium heat until the vinegar starts to evaporate and the sauce becomes like a paste (around 5-7 minutes).

- Add the coriander, season to taste, mix well, turn off the heat and place a lid on the pan.

- In a small bowl, roughly mash the avocado with a fork, add the lime/lemon juice, lightly season and mix thoroughly.

- To serve, spoon the sauce onto a warmed plate, place

the chicken fillets, finely sliced on top and finally the avocado.

- Lightly dust with chilli powder.

Tofu Towers

makes 1 serving

I can't remember where the inspiration for this recipe came from but aubergine, tofu and spices are a great combination and the runny egg completes the dish beautifully.

Ingredients
1 tablespoon sesame seeds
2 slices firm tofu (2-3cm thick)
1 tablespoon sweet chilli sauce
½ level teaspoon ground ginger
½ teaspoon coconut oil
½ teaspoon soy sauce
2 thick slices aubergine
Olive oil
Sea salt and freshly ground black pepper
1-2 large eggs
2 large handfuls fresh spinach leaves

Method
- Toss the sesame seeds in a pan over a medium heat until toasted and set aside (don't take your eye off them as they burn very quickly).

- Wrap the tofu slices in kitchen paper and press firmly to absorb most of the water.

- Mix the chilli sauce, ginger, coconut oil and soy sauce and paint both sides of the tofu slices then put them under a hot grill or on a griddle pan. Cook, turning regularly until they are nicely browned.

- Coat both sides of the aubergine slices with oil and

season with salt and pepper before grilling or griddling as per the tofu. Turn regularly until cooked through and nut brown on both sides.

- Keep the aubergine and tofu warm while you poach the eggs.

- Quickly rinse the spinach leaves, microwave or steam until just wilting then dry the leaves in plenty of kitchen paper.

- To serve, put the aubergine slices on a warmed plate followed by the tofu, the spinach, the sesame seeds and finally the poached eggs.

- If you are merely peckish, one poached egg will suffice. If hungry, opt for two.

Aromatic Lamb/Beef Stew

makes 2 generous or 3 smaller servings

It's all about the long, slow cooking here. Even those who have an issue with 'healthy' alternatives love this stew and it's even better if you leave it in the fridge for a day or freeze and bring it back to the table. Careful though, the temptation to mop up the juices with crusty bread can be hard to control!

Ingredients
2 tablespoons sesame seeds
400g lean lamb or beef, trimmed and cut into bite-sized pieces
Lamb/beef stock
1 small onion, peeled and finely chopped
1 level tablespoon coconut oil
¼ teaspoon saffron
¼ teaspoon ground ginger
½ teaspoon ground coriander
½ teaspoon ground cinnamon

Sea salt and freshly ground black pepper
1 tablespoon Manuka honey (optional)

Method

- Toast the sesame seeds in a dry frying pan, tossing until golden then set aside (watch them as they burn very quickly).

- Put the meat in a medium-sized pan, barely cover with stock and add the onion, oil, saffron, ginger, coriander and cinnamon.

- Stir well, bring to the boil, cover the pan and simmer very gently until the meat is very tender and the liquid has become a rich sauce (about 2 hours but check after an hour and a half and add more stock if necessary).

- Season to taste, stir in the honey (if using) and simmer for a further 5 minutes.

- Cool and refrigerate/freeze at this stage if desired.

- Garnish with toasted sesame seeds before serving.

Spicy Meatball Soup

makes 3 generous or 4 small servings

This soup is taken from our **Soup Can Make You Thin** diet and was so popular we included it in the **Soup Can Make You Thin Cookbook**. There are quite a few ingredients and it does take a little time but boy is it worth it! Play around with the meatballs, make your favourites and refrigerate/freeze ahead and the soup can be made pretty quickly.

Ingredients

For the meatballs:
100g lean minced beef, lamb, pork, chicken or turkey
1 medium egg, lightly whisked
1 tablespoon fresh herbs, finely chopped (parsley/oregano/

thyme/marjoram)
½ teaspoon salt
A few good grindings of black pepper
Small pinch chilli powder

For the soup:
1 tablespoon olive oil
1 small onion, peeled and finely chopped
1 medium-sized carrot, peeled and finely diced
½ celery stalk, peeled and finely sliced
½ red chilli, deseeded and finely diced
1 small clove garlic, peeled and crushed
½ courgette, sliced or chopped
1 level tablespoon tomato puree
600ml beef/lamb/chicken/vegetable stock (depending on your choice of meat)
200g tinned, chopped tomatoes
50g curly kale/savoy cabbage, very finely sliced
Sea salt and freshly ground black pepper
Good handful fresh parsley, chopped

Method
- Thoroughly mix the minced meat, half the whisked egg, herbs, salt, pepper and chilli powder in a bowl with a fork.

- Make around 8 bite-sized meatballs with your hands, lay them on a dish, cover and put in the fridge while you make the soup.

- Heat the oil in a soup pot, add the onion, carrot and celery and saute gently until the onion is soft and translucent and the carrots are slightly tender (don't let the onions brown).

- Add the chilli, garlic, courgette and tomato puree, stir well and saute for a further 5 minutes.

- Add the stock and tomatoes, bring slowly to the boil, reduce the heat and simmer for 15 minutes or until the carrots are tender.

- Add the kale/cabbage and simmer for a further 5 minutes.

- Add the meatballs to the soup with a large spoon and simmer gently until they are cooked through (around 8-10 minutes).

- Check the seasoning and serve; 3-4 meatballs to a bowl, topped with lots of fresh parsley.

Parsley Soup with Chicken Nuggets

makes 1 generous or 2 small servings

This has become a great favourite with our soup fans. It is crazily-green, bursting with goodness and makes a great 'to go' soup if you flask it. You can also top it with other grilled meats, tofu croutons or toasted nuts and seeds for a bit of variety.

Ingredients
2 tablespoons olive oil
1 small onion, peeled and finely sliced/chopped
1 small courgette, cleaned and diced
1 x 28g pack parsley, washed, stalks separated and leaves roughly shredded
1 small clove garlic, peeled and sliced/crushed
400ml chicken or vegetable stock
1 small bay leaf
Salt and pepper
1 small skinless chicken breast, chopped into bite-sized nuggets

Method

- Warm 1 tablespoon of the oil in a soup pot, add the onion and courgette and gently saute until tender but not coloured.

- Add the parsley stalks and garlic and continue to saute for a further 5 minutes.

- Add the stock and bay leaf, bring to the boil, reduce the heat and simmer until the onions and courgette are soft.

- Add the parsley leaves, bring back just to the boil then remove the pot from the heat.

- Remove the bay leaf then transfer the soup to a blender and blitz until very smooth.

- If it is a little too thick for your liking, add more stock or boiling water.

- Strain into a clean pot, check the seasoning and keep on a low heat until ready to serve.

- Put the remaining tablespoon of oil, a good pinch of salt and a few grindings of black pepper in a bowl, add the chicken nuggets and stir until they are well-coated, transfer to a baking sheet lined with tinfoil and grill under a medium heat, turning regularly until slightly crisp on the outside but still juicy inside.

- Drain on kitchen or greaseproof paper, ladle the soup into bowls and top generously with the nuggets.

Mackerel Magic

makes 1 serving

Mackerel has a relatively strong flavour (particularly the smoked variety) so the light, fresh taste of cucumber creates a perfect balance. You are likely to have some sauce left over but it is keeps for a few days in the fridge and works well with a salad or in a lettuce wrap.

Ingredients
16 blanched almonds
100g cucumber, peeled and cut into chunks
1 clove garlic, peeled
10 sprigs dill (stalks removed)
2 tablespoons freshly grated Parmesan cheese
3 tablespoons lemon juice
3 tablespoons olive oil
1 tablespoon sweet chilli sauce
1 mackerel fillet (fresh or smoked)
Sea salt and freshly ground black pepper

Method
• Toss the almonds in a dry frying pan over a high heat until golden brown.

• Put the almonds in a food processor and pulse until they are broken up into small niblets then add the cucumber, garlic, dill, cheese, lemon juice, olive oil, sweet chilli sauce, a teaspoon of sea salt and a few good grindings of black pepper and blitz until everything is blended but still has a bit of texture (like crunchy peanut butter) and set aside.

• Pop the mackerel fillet (skin side down) under the grill (medium heat, low shelf) until piping hot and cooked through before transferring to a warm plate and serving with a couple of generous spoonfuls of the cucumber sauce.

Salmon with Roasted Vegetables
makes 1 serving

This works with any 'meaty' fish (salmon, monkfish, halibut, swordfish etc) and whichever vegetables you have in stock.

Be generous with the vegetables as they shrink while roasting and any extras can be refrigerated and served cold with a salad or in a lettuce wrap.

Ingredients
A mix of vegetables, rinsed, peeled and chopped into bite-sized chunks (peppers, leeks, asparagus, sugar snap peas and baby carrots work well together)
1 tablespoon coconut, avocado or olive oil
Sea salt
Cayenne pepper
250ml fish or vegetable stock
1 salmon steak or fillet (skinned)
1 small onion, peeled and finely sliced
1 bay leaf
A good handful of fresh herbs (dill, marjoram, oregano, lemon thyme)
Freshly ground black pepper

Method
- Preheat the oven to 200C/400F/Gas Mark 6.

- Put the prepared vegetables in a bowl, add the oil, a pinch of salt and a good sprinkling of cayenne pepper, mix well then spread evenly on a baking sheet.

- Place on a fairly high shelf in the oven and roast for 20 minutes before turning and giving them another 5-10 minutes or until the vegetables are tender and well-caramelised around the edges.

- Meanwhile, pour the stock into a shallow saute pan, add the onion, bay leaf, herbs, a pinch of salt and a few good grindings of black pepper and bring slowly to the boil.

- Turn the heat to a gentle simmer, place the salmon on top, cover the pan with a lid or foil and cook for 10-15 minutes or until the salmon is cooked to your liking (cut it in half if you are not sure whether it is cooked right through or not - you're not on Masterchef and there are no cameras!)

- To serve, lift the salmon from the pan and serve on a bed of the roasted vegetables.

- You can sieve the delicious cooking liquor and keep it refrigerated for a couple of days for using with other fish dishes or the fish broth (or just sup it on its own whilst it is still hot - it's that good!)

Mexican-Style Omelette

makes 2 servings

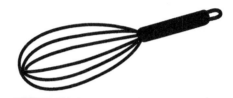

Some can sling a classic omelette together in a matter of minutes, others simply refuse to go there (half a dozen eggs can end up in the bin all too often!) Baking an omelette is the answer for those of us who feel a bit challenged. This is a tasty combo but feel free to sling in whatever is in the fridge, freezer or cupboard.

Ingredients
5cm piece chorizo, finely sliced
A knob of butter
1 small onion, peeled and finely sliced
½ long thin red pepper, de-seeded and finely sliced
6 brown-capped mushrooms, stalks removed, cleaned and finely sliced
2 medium-sized, ripe tomatoes
6 medium eggs
2 tablespoons grated goats cheddar or hard ewes milk cheese

Sea salt and freshly ground black pepper

Method
- Preheat the oven to 200C/400F/Gas Mark 6.

- Skin your tomatoes by putting them in a heat-proof bowl or jar, pouring boiling water over, counting slowly to 30 then draining them - works every time, the skins slip off easily as long as they are ripe.

- Remove the core and seeds from the tomatoes, discard and chop the flesh roughly.

- Place the chorizo in a medium-sized, non-stick oven-proof saute pan and cook over a low heat, turning regularly until the slices release their oils. Lift the chorizo out with a slotted spoon, wrap in a few sheets of kitchen paper to mop up the excess oil and set aside.

- Add a knob of butter to the pan and once melted add the onions and peppers and cook over a low heat until soft.

- Add the mushrooms, turn the heat up and stir briskly until the mushrooms, onions and pepper are slightly caramelised at the edges.

- Turn the heat back down to low, add the tomato and chorizo, mix well and allow everything to continue at a very low simmer.

- Lightly beat the eggs in a bowl, add a good pinch of salt and a few grindings of black pepper, mix well and pour into the pan.

- Make sure the egg covers everything (push the other ingredients down into the liquid) then transfer to the middle of the oven and bake, uncovered for 5 minutes.

- Remove the pan from the oven, turn on the grill, scatter the cheese on top of the omelette, place the pan on a low shelf, keep an eye on it and when the cheese is nicely

73

browned and bubbling turn the heat off.

- Transfer to a warmed serving plate (a fish slice or spatula helps here!)

- This recipe serves 2 but if you are eating 'solo', put the other half in the fridge and have it cold the next day (or the day after) with a salad.

RECIPES
(starch days)

Nutty Bircher Muesli

makes 1 generous or 2 smaller servings

I learned how to make real authentic Bircher muesli whilst working as a waitress in the mountains of Switzerland in my early 20s. Since then, I have been playing around with the revered Dr Maximilian Bircher-Benner's classic, restorative recipe and this is one that doesn't include fruit but still has a wonderfully sweet edge.

Ingredients
6 tablespoons oats
140ml coconut water
2 tablespoons flaked almonds (toasted or un-toasted)
½ tablespoon Manuka honey
1 tablespoon 0% fat Greek yoghurt
2 teaspoons lemon/lime juice
½ apple, peeled, cored and grated
4 fresh mint leaves, very finely chopped

Method
- Combine all the ingredients in a bowl, mix really well, cover and place in the fridge overnight.

- Serve with a sprinkling of cinnamon powder or grated nutmeg on top.

Scrambled Eggs on Hot Buttered Toast

makes 1 serving

Why, on a starch day would you have cereals when you can have delectably-creamy scrambled eggs on hot buttered toast - beats me!

Ingredients
2 large eggs
Sea salt and freshly ground black pepper
1 large or 2 small slices dark brown 'chewy' bread
Butter
Extras: smoked salmon, ham, grated hard cheese, chives, herbs

Method
- Have your bread ready in the toaster or ready to go under a hot grill.

- Put a small non-stick pan over a medium heat.

- Lightly beat the eggs in a bowl, season with salt and pepper, pour into the pan and start stirring gently (use a wooden spoon with a pointed end to get to the very edges of the pan).

- Keep scrambling until three-quarters of the egg is a creamy mass then turn off the heat.

- Toast the bread.

- Add 'extras' to the pan if using and keep stirring until there is no liquid egg left.

- Quickly butter your toast, top with the scrambled egg and dig in.

Light Chicken Broth

makes 3 generous or 4 small servings

There is not much I can say about this chicken soup other than that it feeds much, much more than the soul! My best friend and trusted soup guru, Jean threw this one together one evening when she had a few chicken thighs that were nearing their use-by date and the rest is now history. Trust me, you could live on this soup for 2 weeks and never get bored with it!

Ingredients
2 chicken thighs, skin on
1 tablespoon olive or avocado oil
2 stalks celery, peeled and finely sliced
1 small onion, peeled and finely sliced
1 small carrot, peeled and finely diced
600ml chicken stock
40g brown rice
1 teaspoon horseradish sauce
A generous bunch of parsley, stalks removed and leaves very finely chopped
Sea salt and freshly ground black pepper

Method
- Roast the chicken pieces in a medium to hot oven until the skins are crisp and the flesh is cooked through while you make the soup.

- Warm the oil in a soup pot, add the celery, onion and carrot and saute gently until the vegetables are tender (about 15 minutes).

- Add the stock and bring slowly to the boil.

- Reduce the heat, add the rice and simmer, covered until the rice is cooked (around 20 minutes).

- Skin the chicken pieces and shred/chop the flesh before adding to the soup with the horseradish sauce and parsley.

- Stir well and season to taste.

- As rice soaks up a lot of liquid, you will probably have to add more stock or water to achieve the light, brothy experience if you are not supping this soup immediately and have refrigerated/frozen it for future use.

Spinach and Watercress Soup

makes 2 generous or 3 small servings

Boy, is this soup green but boy is it special and the addition of the oats, lemon juice and lemon zest make it a protein-rich, antioxidant, vitamin and mineral-rich elixir that is quite the most delicious cure in a bowl.

Ingredients
1 tablespoon olive oil
1 small onion, peeled and finely chopped
500ml chicken or vegetable stock
1 level tablespoon porridge oats
1 x 75g bag spinach leaves
½ x 75g bag watercress
1 tablespoon fresh lemon juice
Salt salt and freshly ground black pepper

Method

- Warm the oil in a soup pot and saute the onion gently until soft.

- Add the stock and the porridge oats, bring slowly to the boil, turn down the heat and simmer for 15 minutes.

- Add the spinach and watercress and keep stirring whilst bringing the soup back to the boil then turn off the heat.

- Blend the whole lot until you have a smooth, foamy soup then return to a clean pan.

- Heat through gently, add the lemon juice, season to taste and serve.

- You can grate a little lemon zest on top of each bowl for added zing.

Crispy-Topped Baked Fish, Chicken or Tofu

makes 1 serving

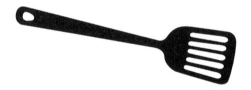

How do you turn a dull dish into a tasty dish? Give it a topping! Get into the habit of making this topping (which can be made ahead and refrigerated or frozen), put in a little more or less of any of the ingredients or experiment and you can sharpen up just about any meat, poultry, fish, shellfish or vegetarian dish.

Ingredients
1 white fish fillet **or**
1 slice of tofu (around 2cm thick) **or**

1 medium-sized skinless chicken breast
1 tablespoon oats
1 tablespoon fresh parsley, finely chopped
1 tablespoon lemon juice
Sea salt and freshly ground black pepper
2 teaspoons olive or coconut oil
3 spring onions, trimmed and finely sliced
2 heaped teaspoons tomato puree
1 medium-sized tomato, sliced
15g Parmesan cheese, grated

Method
- Preheat the oven to 200C/400F/Gas Mark 6.

- In a small bowl, mix the oats, parsley and lemon juice, lightly season and set aside.

- Warm the oil in a small saute pan and cook the spring onions over a medium heat until soft then add the tomato puree and mix well.

- **For fish or tofu:** Place a sheet of baking foil in a small oven-proof dish, place the fish or tofu in the middle and pull up the sides of the foil so you create an open-topped parcel.

- Top the fish/tofu with the spring onion/tomato puree mix, arrange the tomato slices on top and finally the oat mix (don't close the parcel) then place the dish on a middle shelf in the oven and bake until cooked through.

- Thin fish fillets and tofu will take around 5-6 minutes, thicker/denser fish fillets will take around 8-12 minutes. Have a peek and check that the fish flakes nicely and the juice is clear.

- Remove from the oven, turn the oven off and the grill on (to a medium heat), scatter the cheese on top, grill on the lowest shelf until the cheese melts and is just beginning to brown (around 5 minutes) then with a fish slice, lift the fish/tofu onto a warmed serving plate and spoon over the cooking juices.

- **For the chicken:** Place the chicken on the foil, lightly season, add a splash of oil, scrunch the foil so it creates a loose but sealed parcel and bake for 10 minutes then open up the parcel, top as per the fish/tofu and bake for a further 10 minutes or until the juices run clear and the chicken is cooked through.

- Continue as before and serve.

Perfect Overnight Porridge

makes 1 large or 2 smaller servings

The fabulous thing about porridge is that there is no definitive recipe or cooking method - it's more of a personal thing. I am a Scot and over nearly 60 years have sampled many a bowl of porridge - some which take your breath away, some which glue your gums together and some which are way too thin and watery! Here's one of my fat-busting favourites where you soak the oats overnight so it takes less time to cook, is quickly ready to scoff or can be transport in a wide-necked vacuum flask.

Ingredients
1 teacup medium-cut oats
3 teacups hot but not boiling water
Decent pinch of salt

Method
- Place the water in a heat-proof bowl and gradually but meaningfully whisk in the oats - you don't want any clumps.

- Leave to cool a little then cover the bowl and place in the refrigerator overnight.

- In the morning, transfer the porridge to a non-stick pan

and cook over a medium heat until bubbling, stirring all the time.

- Add the salt and continue to stir for another few minutes – if it is a little thick for your liking, just add some boiling water.

- Serve with a spoonful or two of double cream, a drizzle of runny honey and a good sprinkling of cinnamon powder or grated nutmeg.

If you forgot to put the porridge in the refrigerator overnight, the whole exercise will just take a little longer. Put the water in a small non-stick pan over a medium heat, add the oatmeal in a slow but steady stream and stir enthusiastically until bubbling noisily. Add the salt and continue cooking and stirring for another 5 minutes before serving as above.

Thai Curry Sweet Potato Soup

makes 2 generous or 3 small servings

If you like a bit of spice in your life (remember, spices are fat burners) this will likely become a classic in your repertoire. This is a tasty and filling soup which you can play around with - hotter in winter, cooler in summer, it's another of Jean's triumphs!

Ingredients
125g sweet potato peeled and chopped into bite-sized chunks
½ long, thin red pepper, de-seeded and cut into fine strips
½ x 400ml tin coconut milk (not 'low fat' as it is liable to split when heated)
200ml chicken or vegetable stock
1 teaspoon Thai Red Curry Paste
6 fresh or frozen raw prawns **or**
1 small skinless chicken breast cut into long, thin strips **or**
A dozen cubes of firm tofu, drained and dried

20g fresh basil leaves, chopped or torn (also works well with baby spinach leaves)

Method

- Put the sweet potato, red pepper, coconut milk, stock and Thai Red Curry Paste into a soup pot, stir well and bring slowly to the boil.

- Reduce the heat and simmer very gently for 20 minutes or until the sweet potato is tender and just beginning to fall apart, this will thicken the soup.

- Add the prawns, chicken or tofu and stir over a very low heat to cook through. The prawns and tofu will only take a couple of minutes, the chicken slightly longer.

- Stir in the basil leaves and when just wilted, serve the soup.

- You can add more Thai Red Curry Paste before adding the protein if you like a bit more spice.

Warm Salad with Haggis

makes 2 servings

I am in the fortunate position of knowing and occasionally working with Jo Macsween, the driving force behind Macsween of Edinburgh www.macsween.co.uk who, in my view make simply the best haggis in the world. She recently published **The Macsween Haggis Bible**, a delightful little book which addresses haggis mysteries, quashes a few haggis myths and offers an inspiring selection of recipes which show haggis off to its very best. Here's one that ticks a whole load of fat busting boxes!

Ingredients
3 heaped teaspoons coarse grain mustard
6 tablespoons extra virgin cold-pressed olive oil
1 tablespoon white wine vinegar

Sea salt
Freshly ground black pepper
1 x 130g packet 'microwave in 60 seconds' traditional or
vegetarian haggis
100g baby salad leaves
½ Granny Smith apple, peeled, cored and finely diced
50g red onion, peeled and very finely sliced

Method
- To make the mustard dressing, whisk the mustard and vinegar together, blend in the oil, season and put to one side.

- Heat the haggis in the microwave, arrange the salad leaves on the plates, gently pour over the dressing, break up the haggis, place on top of the leaves and garnish with the apple and red onion.

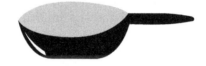

Mince and Mash

makes 2 servings

Mince and potatoes can't be beat when it comes to comfort food and I may well be the first nutritionist ever to recommend it in a super fast fat loss plan! But why not? Good quality protein, rich in iron and other health-giving nutrients, filling and satisfying, downright delicious and cooked this way, waistline-friendly - what's not to love?

Ingredients
250g very lean beef or lamb mince
1 small onion, peeled and finely chopped
2 heaped teaspoons cornflour

250ml beef or lamb stock
Sea salt and freshly ground black pepper
1 tablespoon Worcestershire sauce
500g mashing potatoes, peeled and cut into even sized chunks
25g of butter (optional)

Method

- Heat a non-stick pan over a high heat, add the mince and using a wooden fork or spatula, brown the mince, separating all the mince morsels along the way.

- Add the onion and continue to stir over a high heat until everything has a nicely-browned edge, add the cornflour, mix in well then turn the heat down a little.

- Add the stock, stir until the liquid absorbs the cornflour, add the Worcestershire sauce, a good pinch of salt and a few grindings of black pepper, bring to the boil, stirring continuously then turn the heat down to a very gentle simmer, put the lid on and cook for 45 minutes.

- After 45 minutes, remove the lid, turn the heat up to medium and let the mince bubble away and thicken.

- Meanwhile, put the potato chunks in a pot, pour boiling water over to just cover, add a good pinch of salt, bring to the boil then turn the heat down, put a lid on and cook for around 20 minutes or until the potatoes are tender but not falling apart.

- When the potatoes are cooked, drain and cover with a tea towel for a few minutes to absorb some of the steam before returning to the pan, adding the butter (if using) and mashing furiously until wonderfully-smooth and creamy.

- I like the mash on the bottom and the mince on top so the gravy seeps into the mash but feel free to do your own thing!

Rice and Stuff

makes 2 generous servings

Not a very elegant title, I admit but when it comes to making a filling, nutritious and fat busting dish which includes rice, there 'aint many rules! When you have been 'starch-free' for a few days you can get the rice out of the cupboard and add all sorts as long as you remember to include some protein. Here's one suggestion.

Ingredients
1 tablespoon olive oil
A knob of butter
1 small onion, peeled and finely chopped
4 spring onions, trimmed and finely sliced
1 clove garlic, peeled and finely chopped
½ medium courgette, diced
1 'beef' mushroom, stem removed, peeled and roughly chopped
4 tablespoons brown basmati rice
4 thin slices prociutto crudo or Parma ham, roughly chopped
12 tablespoons boiling water
1 tablespoon dried mixed herbs
Sea salt and freshly ground black pepper
1 x 200g can chopped tomatoes
2 good handfuls fresh spinach leaves

Method
- Preheat oven to 190°C/375°F/Gas Mark 5.

- Place a non-stick oven-proof pan or casserole dish over a medium heat, warm the oil and butter then add the onion and saute until soft.

- Add the spring onion and garlic and continue to saute for a further 5 minutes.

- Turn up the heat, add the courgette and mushrooms and

stir until everything starts to slightly brown around the edges (3-5 minutes).

- Add the rice and ham, stir well so everything is well-combined, pour in the boiling water, add the mixed herbs, season and when bubbling nicely, turn off the heat, put the lid on (or cover with kitchen foil) and transfer to the oven.

- Bake for 30 minutes then test to see if the rice is cooked to your liking. If all the liquid has been absorbed but the rice still needs a little more cooking, add another few tablespoons of boiling water and return to the oven for another 10 minutes then check again.

- When the rice is cooked and all the liquid has been absorbed, remove the pan to the hob, use a fork to separate the rice grains then add the tomatoes and spinach and stir briskly over a medium heat until the spinach is just wilted then check the seasoning and serve.

Fragrant Chicken Casserole

makes 2 generous or 3 small servings

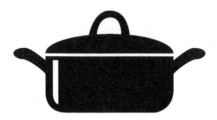

The blitzed paste that forms the basis of this recipe works well not only with chicken but also with turkey, meaty fish like monkfish and halibut and shellfish. If you have time, make the paste ahead of time and refrigerate or freeze and if you add more liquid to the casserole you can turn it into a soup - endless possibilities!

Ingredients

1 red chilli, deseeded and roughly chopped
3 shallots, peeled and roughly chopped
2 cloves garlic, peeled
3cm piece of fresh ginger, peeled and roughly chopped
1 heaped teaspoon lemon grass paste
½ teaspoon ground turmeric
½ teaspoon ground coriander
1 tablespoon fresh parsley or coriander leaves
1 tablespoon olive oil
½ x 400ml tin coconut milk
50ml chicken stock
1 large or 2 small skinless chicken breasts, sliced into strips
50g thin cooked rice noodles
Sea salt and freshly ground black pepper
Juice of half a lime

Method

- Blitz the chillies, shallots, garlic, ginger, lemongrass, ground turmeric, ground coriander, fresh parsley/coriander and oil in a food processor or spice mixer until you have a rough paste.

- Transfer to a medium-sized pot and cook over a very gentle heat for 8-10 minutes.

- Add the coconut milk and stock, bring just to the boil, reduce the heat to its lowest setting and simmer for 10 minutes.

- Add the chicken and simmer, stirring for a further 5 minutes until the chicken strips are cooked through..

- Add the noodles and slowly bring back to just boiling.

- Turn off the heat, season to taste, add the lime juice and let the casserole stand for a couple of minutes before serving.

MY BOOKS, BLOGS Etc

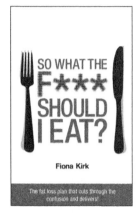

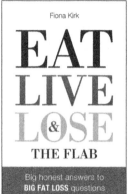

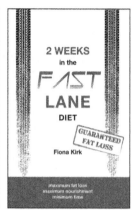

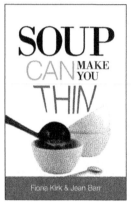

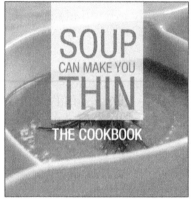

www.fatbustforever.com

www.souperydupery.com

www.facebook.com/fionakirkbooks

www.twitter.com/FatBustForever

www.pinterest.com/fionakirkbooks

WEBSITES, BLOGS & CONTACTS

Nutritional Therapy

If you have an underlying health condition which may be affecting your ability to lose weight, suspect you may be intolerant to certain foods or merely wish to ascertain which diet or supplement programme is best for you, a consultation with a qualified practitioner could be the answer. Go to www.bant.org.uk and click 'Find a Local Practitioner'. Members of the British Association for Applied Nutrition and Nutritional Therapy offer the very highest standards of integrity, knowledge, competence and professional practice. The majority of BANT members are based in the UK but there are also a number practicing in other parts of the world. Wherever you are, ensure that any practitioner you decide to consult holds a recognised professional qualification and has a minimum of 3 years relevant training.

Should you wish to learn more about nutritional therapy you can embark on a home study course with The Institute for Optimum Nutrition www.ion.ac.uk where you can also sign up for their regular newsletters and/or subscribe to the monthly magazine and keep up to date with the latest nutrition research news.

Diet/Motivational Websites and Blogs

A small but inspiring selection of some I follow:

www.marksdailyapple.com

www.beyondveg.com

www.mercola.com

www.thefooddoctor.com

www.zoeharcombe.com

www.drbriffa.com

www.petecohen.com

www.fightingfifty.co.uk

www.londonmumsmagazine.com

Food Blogs

Being a real foodie with a passion for ever-more input, my list of favourites is very long but here are a few that never disappoint! Also, click on some of the blogs they follow - bloggers are a very selective bunch!

www.sweetpotatochronicles.com

www.smittenkitchen.com

www.veganyumyum.com

www.101cookbooks.com

www.mycustardpie.com

www.deliciouslyella.com

www.lemonsandanchovies.com

www.anjasfood4thought.com

www.mydarlinglemonthyme.com

www.sweetpaulmag.com/eat.htm

www.thedeliciouslife.com

COPYRIGHT

2 Weeks in the Super Fast Lane.
Copyright © 2014 by Fiona Kirk

Note to Readers
If you are pregnant, breastfeeding, on regular medication, have concerns about your health or are under the age of 16 you should consult your doctor or health practitioner before embarking on any new eating programme. Every effort has been made to present the information in this book in a clear, complete and accurate manner, however not every situation can be anticipated and the information in this book cannot take the place of a medical analysis of individual health needs. The author hereby disclaims any and all liability resulting from injuries or damage caused by following any recommendations in this book.

Design and layout: **Milkbar Creative**
ISBN 978 0 9929106 0 0

CPSIA information can be obtained at www.ICGtesting.com
Printed in the USA
LVOW04s0014070315

429549LV00035B/2348/P